The Fertility Awareness Handbook

Barbara Kass-Annese was born in Ohio. She received her Nursing Diploma from Kent State University and her Nurse Practitioner training in Family Planning and Gynecology through the Boston Family Planning Project and the University of California at Los Angeles. She followed this with educational programs at leading U.S. hospitals, including Harvard Medical School and New York University Medical School.

Ms. Kass-Annese currently works in a private women's health care practice, subspecializing in infertility. She often conducts seminars for colleges and hospitals, and appears on radio and television to discuss healthcare topics such as human sexuality, fertility awareness, and natural family planning aids to conception and contraception.

Hal C. Danzer was born in Montana, and moved with his family to southern California where he completed his schooling. He graduated from St. Louis University School of Medicine, and returned to Los Angeles to intern at the L.A. County–U.S.C. Medical Center. He later completed his residency in Obstetrics and Gynecology, followed by a Fellowship in Reproductive Endocrinology, at Cedars-Sinai Medical Center.

Dr. Danzer is currently active in both education and research. He has served as an investigator for one of the largest studies of Natural Family Planning, and continues to teach at UCLA. He also maintains a private practice, subspecializing in infertility and reproductive endocrinology.

The
FERTILITY
AWARENESS
HANDBOOK

The
Natural Guide
to
Avoiding
or
Achieving
Pregnancy

BARBARA KASS-ANNESE, R.N., C.N.P.
&
HAL C. DANZER, M.D.

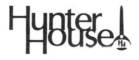

This is a completely revised edition of the "The Fertility Awareness Workbook" first published in 1981 as "Patterns" (ISBN 0-941304-02-7) by Patterns Publishing, Redondo Beach, CA, and later issued by G.P. Putnam's Sons, New York, NY; Printed Matter, Inc., Atlanta, GA; and Hunter House Inc., Publishers. This edition published in 1992 by Hunter House Inc., Publishers.

Library of Congress Cataloging-in-Publication Data
Kass-Annese, Barbara.
The fertility awareness handbook /
Barbara Kass-Annese & Hal Danzer. — 6th ed.
p. cm.
Updated ed. of: The fertility awareness workbook. 5th ed. 1990.
Includes bibliographical references and index.
ISBN 0-89793-096-7 : $11.95
1. Natural family planning. 2. Fertility, Human. I. Danzer, Hal. II. Kass-Annese, Barbara. Fertility awareness workbook. III. Title.
RG136.5.K37   1992
613.9'4—dc20   91-44714

Original illustrations by Tom Rachel, revised by Sparrow Fraenkel
Book design by Qalagraphia, cover design by Theresa Smith
Set in Cheltenham by 847 Communications, Alameda, CA
Production manager: Paul J. Frindt
Editorial coordination by Corrine M. Sahli and Lisa Lee
Publisher: Kiran S. Rana

Manufactured in the United States of America
9 8 7 6 5 4 3 2   6th edition

Contents

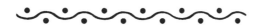

Acknowledgments

The authors express their thanks to:
John Altamura
Bart Andrews
Joe Bectol
Dana Chalberg
Blake Conway
Gareth Esersky
Michelle Martino
H. Roy Matlen
F. Clyde Petersen
Kiran Rana
Sherri Robb
Barbara S. Rollins
who made *THE FERTILITY AWARENESS HANDBOOK* and its
predecessors, *THE FERTILITY AWARENESS WORKBOOK* and
PATTERNS, possible.

Introduction

Are there times when you have been mystified by your own body and reproductive organs and feel that you should have been told more?

Did you know . . . that a woman can become pregnant *only* during *a few days* of each menstrual cycle?

Did you know . . . that a woman may become pregnant on Friday from having intercourse on Monday?

Did you know . . . that having intercourse during menstrual bleeding can sometimes lead to pregnancy?

Do you want . . . a safe and effective alternative to the hormonal, spermicidal and mechanical methods of birth control?

Did you know . . . there are natural ways that are safe and effective in preventing pregnancy that can also be an aid for achieving pregnancy?

The Fertility Awareness Handbook will help you to know more, to no longer be mystified about your body and reproduction.

It has been written for those who want a greater understanding of their bodies. *It is not only a book about preventing and achieving pregnancy, but also a book for those who want to learn what is normal and healthy for them.*

This book will explain and illustrate the most up-to-date information about women's and men's reproductive systems. It focuses on the naturally occurring changes that take place within a woman's body. These changes, called fertility signs, can be used to determine the days during each menstrual cycle when a woman can and cannot become pregnant.

Knowledge about fertility signs has existed for some time but has not been widely available until now. This book was designed to provide you with this knowledge—knowledge that can be used in many rewarding ways throughout your life.

All of nature is made of patterns, as a woven fabric is made of patterns of threads, one overlapping the other, creating an intricate tapestry.

The seasons represent patterns of nature, each leading slowly and fittingly into the next.

Our bodies, like the seasons, also have patterns. Our youth slips inevitably into adolescence, into adulthood, then into middle-age, and finally into the later years. During this lifecycle our bodies reveal various patterns to us.

The set of patterns that we concentrate on in this book—the patterns of fertility—can be thought of as a special language of the woman's body. *The Fertility Awareness Handbook* will show you how to understand this language.

It provides accurate information about reproduction and includes revealing information about a woman's body. It also provides specific instruction on the use of two methods of family planning:

1. Natural Family Planning, and

2. Fertility Awareness Method

The Fertility Awareness Handbook has a clear logic to it. It begins with a brief history of natural family planning, followed by basic chapters on how the reproductive systems of women and men work. If you are to understand the body's language about fertility, then you should first learn exactly why the reproductive organs work the way they do. All of this basic knowledge is meant to help you increase your awareness of the normal and natural changes of the reproductive cycle.

Following the chapters on basics, there is a detailed explanation and description of the body's special language—*fertility signs.* Knowing exactly what fertility signs are and how they work, as well as why they work, will give you confidence with your own personal method of family planning.

Because some couples experience difficulty achieving a pregnancy, the subject of infertility and instructions on how to use fertility signs to increase the possibility of pregnancy are discussed next.

The next section gives step-by-step instructions on how to observe and record your fertility signs and how to prevent pregnancy. The book closes with a discussion of the natural family planning and fertility awareness methods, their advantages and disadvantages.

As you begin reading about the facts of fertility awareness and end with considering your own feelings, we hope you find this awareness and information rewarding and enriching.

Chapter 1

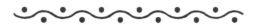

Natural Family Planning and Fertility Awareness Methods: What Are They?

Almost everywhere you turn, you see and hear references to the word *natural*—natural food, natural childbirth, natural lifestyles.

We also want to use the word *natural* in this original meaning—that which occurs in nature, like the natural workings of the human body. So when we say that you have natural information, we mean that your body actually does offer the signs we talk about, signs that are based on accurate, specific, and available natural body language. They are called *fertility signs*.

BODY SIGNS = FERTILITY SIGNS

Proper use of fertility awareness will let you know your *fertile days*—those days during the month when it is possible to become pregnant. Since you are able to know your fertile days, you will also know those days during the month when you cannot become pregnant. These are called the *infertile days*.

If a pregnancy is being planned, then your having intercourse during fertile days offers the very highest possibility—the maximum chance—to become pregnant.

Natural family planning (NFP) is the name for various methods of family planning that, when used for pregnancy prevention, combine the use of fertility signs and abstinence from intercourse during fertile days.

Fertility awareness method (FAM) is a family planning method also. Both methods use the same naturally occurring fertility signs to guide you. However, with FAM, instead of abstaining from intercourse, you can choose to use a cervical cap, a diaphragm, contraceptive sponge, a condom, and/or a spermicide during the fertile days.

In other words, FAM teaches you how to identify the few days during each menstrual cycle when some form of contraception needs to be used. Because some people find abstinence during the fertile days unacceptable to them, FAM offers a way to develop understanding about fertility and how to use this understanding to meet one's family planning needs.

Regardless of whether NFP or FAM is used, the significant point is this: your body reveals fertility signs that enable you to identify the fertile and infertile days during each menstrual cycle and all of this is based on a natural language that is spoken by your body.

By learning this language, you can join the thousands of women and men who are now enjoying these alternative approaches to family planning!

Chapter 2

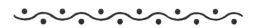

A Bit of History

Since the beginning of recorded history the desire for reliable methods to prevent pregnancy and enhance fertility has existed. Women beyond the healthy childbearing years or women who were ill were not expected to bear children. The woman who experienced repeated stillbirths or very difficult deliveries often sought to avoid future pregnancies. Times of war, famine, or inability to adequately provide for the health and safety of a child were also important factors in the choice to delay pregnancy. As you can see from these examples, people throughout the ages had many of the same reasons for pregnancy prevention as we do today.

HOW HAVE PEOPLE ATTEMPTED
TO PREVENT PREGNANCY?

Beginning with pre-Biblical times, people have used abstinence, breastfeeding, withdrawal, magical potions, charms, and herbal mixtures to prevent pregnancy.

During the time of the ancient Hebrews, one method used was a spongy substance placed inside the vagina to block sperm. Greek and Roman literature tells us of many methods of birth control, including tying up asparagus to be worn as a charm, and vaginal suppositories made from honey and peppermint juice.

During the Middle Ages in Europe and Islam a number of recipes, many magical, were used to avoid pregnancy. One unusual recipe instructed a woman who did not want to become pregnant

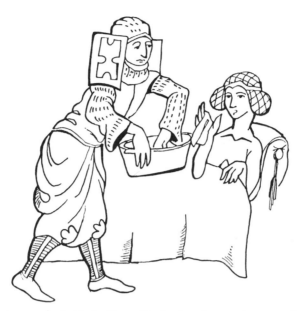

to soak a piece of cloth in the oil of a barberry tree and place it on the left side of her forehead. Another method suggested eating beans on an empty stomach and rubbing tar on the penis prior to intercourse as forms of birth control. A Moroccan ritual made use of a ring containing a special stone set in gold or silver. The man wore this ring during intercourse. If pregnancy was to be avoided, he would turn the ring so that the stone faced one of his fingers. In North Africa some tribal women ate a piece of honeycomb mixed with a few dead bees and placed between pieces of bread. Some Sumatran women placed a small ball of opium inside their vaginas.

A folk belief of Southern Russian women described taking a few drops of their menstrual blood and letting it flow into a hole made in the first egg of a young hen. The woman would bury the egg near a table in the room. The egg was left buried for nine days and nights. When it was removed, the worms found in it were counted. It was believed that the number of worms represented the number of children the woman would have. If she threw the egg into fire, she wouldn't have children. If she desired children, she would throw the egg into water.

Other methods of birth control included douching solutions made of lemon juice and the husks of mahogany nuts, algae, or seaweed placed inside the vagina before intercourse, carrying a child's tooth, and drinking thyme and lavender tea.

Since fertility was usually not understood, it was often considered mystical. Slowly, as a truer understanding about the facts of physiology and reproduction emerged, science and technology began to replace the magical.

Around the middle of the 18th century, although potions and ceremonies continued to be used, modern mechanical forms of birth control began emerging. The condom was one of the first of these to be introduced.

The birth control movement in America had begun by 1828. Techniques included withdrawal, using a vaginal sponge made from sheep's wool or silk, and using douching solutions made from white oak bark, green tea, or vinegar and water. Although the use of the diaphragm emerged in Holland during the early 1880s, it was not introduced to American women until the early 1920s. Between the 1920s and 1930s the rhythm method, Grafenberg intrauterine silver ring, and spermicides began to be used. From that point on several types of intrauterine devices were developed. Finally "the Pill" entered the mainstream of American life during the 1960s.

WHERE DOES NFP FIT INTO ALL OF THIS? WHAT KIND OF HISTORY DOES IT HAVE?

We know historically that in various areas throughout the world women have used and continue to use breastfeeding as a natural means of child spacing. Yet, compared to the thousands of real and "magical" methods of contraception that have evolved and been recorded, little has been written about other forms of natural family planning. There is limited information available about Africans and Native Americans, as well as other groups, who appear to have had some knowledge of their fertility cycles and practiced abstinence from intercourse. It is known that these groups did use one of the major fertility signs, cervical mucus, as a means to achieve or avoid pregnancy, and it is still used by them today.

Over 150 years ago a researcher, Dr. Bischoff, found eggs present in the uterus and fallopian tubes of a female dog while the dog was bleeding—"in heat." Because of this discovery he assumed that women must also have eggs present during their menstrual bleeding. Therefore, he believed that women became pregnant if they had intercourse during their periods. As a result of his findings, a natural birth control schedule was developed. It stated that if pregnancy was to be avoided, intercourse should not occur during the menstrual period, as well as 5 days before it and 9 days after it.[1] It was considered that these were the days when the woman could become pregnant. We now know that just the opposite is true!

This "natural birth control" continued to be practiced until the 1930s, and countless women became pregnant trying to use this totally incorrect information.

However, not all past information was incorrect. As early as 1857, there were descriptions of women who believed they could tell when they were ovulating because once a month they experienced internal aching or a painful feeling in the area of the ovaries. (Ovulation is the release of the egg from the ovary.)

This pain with ovulation continued to be discussed and written about for years. In 1935, Dr. Cyrus Anderson wrote a paper entitled, "Teaching the Patient to Observe Symptoms of Ovulation." This paper discussed ovulation pain and how women could be taught to recognize it.[2]

Ovulation pain, as you will soon learn, can be used by some women as a fertility sign. One of the other fertility signs you will learn about is the temperature of the body at rest, known as basal body temperature. It was studied as early as 1876 by Dr. Marie Putnam Jacobi.[3] She found that the basal body temperature rises and drops at certain points during the menstrual cycle.

Cervical mucus, another fertility sign, was also written about in the 1800s. In fact, around the mid-1800s it was observed that this mucus changed in amount and quality throughout the menstrual cycle. From these observations it was believed that a particular kind of mucus was needed to achieve a pregnancy.

Finally, in 1929, the rhythm method was developed when two men on opposite sides of the world, and working independently of each other, discovered that an egg is released from the ovary approximately 14 days before the next menstrual flow begins. This discovery formed the basis of the Ogina-Knaus Calendar Rhythm Method, named after the two discoverers, Dr. Ogina and Dr. Knaus. However, the rhythm method did not prove accurate enough to be used by all women as a form of birth control. This is because the success of the rhythm method is dependent upon a woman experiencing consistently regular cycles, an uncommon event for many. The life span of the egg and sperm were not then known, which also contributed to the ineffectiveness of the rhythm method.

In 1962, Dr. Hartman found that sperm could live in the woman's body for three days, while the egg lives for one day. This added up to a 4-day period of time during the menstrual cycle when a woman could become pregnant. We now know that if the proper conditions are present in the woman's body, sperm may live and remain capable of fertilizing the egg for a period of 3 to 5 days.

During the 1960s, an Australian team of physicians, Drs. John and Evelyn Billings, conducted extensive research on cervical mucus. They were attempting to find a method of natural family planning that would be more accurate than the rhythm method. Consequently, their research led to the development of the Billings Method, also known as the cervical mucus method or ovulation method. This method is based on using the observations of the cervical mucus to determine the fertile and infertile days of the menstrual cycle.

Even before the development of the Billings Method, a form of the sympto-thermal method of natural family planning was made available. This method is based on the use of the cervical mucus, basal body temperature, and other symptoms of ovulation to determine the days of infertility and fertility.

All this adds up to the fact that reliable methods of natural family planning, the ovulation and sympto-thermal methods, have been used by people throughout the world for over 35 years!

HOW EFFECTIVE ARE THESE METHODS OF NATURAL FAMILY PLANNING?

Before answering this question, it is important to acknowledge that a woman's and man's feelings about pregnancy play a very important part in how a method of birth control is used. Women and men who are motivated to avoid a pregnancy tend to use a method more carefully, and careful use means fewer pregnancies.

Because of this fact and others, effectiveness rates, or how successful a method of birth control is, are discussed in two ways. One is the *theoretical effectiveness* rate. This type of effectiveness rate tells us how well a method works when used perfectly. In other words, no mistakes are made on the parts of the clinician or instructor providing the birth control method or the person using the method. The second type of effectiveness rate is called *use effectiveness*. This is the real effectiveness of the method, taking into account human error made by the user of the method, the clinician, or the instructor.

For example, if a couple using NFP did not abstain during a fertile time and the woman became pregnant, this would be called a user failure. A user failure may also be because of the inability of the couple to understand the method, and this may be due to the teacher, the couple, or a combination of both.

If a couple using NFP perfectly becomes pregnant, this is a theoretical failure, a failure of the method to prevent pregnancy.

A 3-year study, supported by the Department of Health, Education, and Welfare, and completed in 1979 at Cedar-Sinai Medical Center in Los Angeles, compared the effectiveness of the ovulation method and the sympto-thermal method. Over 1200 couples participated in this study. It was found that the ovulation method was approximately 78% effective. This means that 22 out of every 100 women who began use of the method, and who did not stop using it for any reason, became pregnant within one year. The sympto-thermal method was determined to be approximately 89% use effective, which means that out of every 100 women who began use of this method and did not stop using it for any reason, 11 became pregnant within one year. The results of this particular study are generally similar to many others which have been conducted throughout the world.

Many of the pregnancies in this study occurred because people "took chances" and had intercourse during the fertile time, did not understand the use of the methods, or did not follow other instructions necessary for the effective use of these two methods.

The reason why the couples using the sympto-thermal (S-T) method experienced a lower number of pregnancies is not completely understood. However, the Cedar-Sinai study and others, in addition to our own experience in working with these methods, suggest that for many people the S-T method is easier to teach, to learn and to use properly. The findings of this particular study, in addition to many others, have consistently suggested that the theoretical effectiveness rates of both methods are approximately equal. When instructed correctly by the teachers, in combination with the couples' understanding and proper use of the methods, the effectiveness rates are approximately 98%.

The effectiveness rates of the natural family planning methods are comparable with almost all of the other methods of contraception.

	Theoretical Effectiveness	Use Effectiveness
Birth Control Pills	99.66%	90–94%
Condom and Spermicide	99+%	95%
Intrauterine Device	97–99%	95%
Condom	97%	90%
Diaphragm	97%	83%
Spermicidal Foam	97%	78%

THE FERTILITY AWARENESS METHOD HAS AN EVEN BRIEFER HISTORY THAN NATURAL FAMILY PLANNING

Several years ago, groups of professionals active in family planning felt it to be important that women and men have complete information about their fertility patterns, regardless of whether or not they chose to use NFP.

Not only did they feel this information itself could enable people to avoid pregnancy naturally, but they also felt that it could be used in combination with other methods such as the diaphragm, spermicide and condoms. (See the Bibliography if you are interested in learning more about various methods of contraception.) Combining fertility sign information and other methods became known as fertility awareness method (FAM). FAM provides people with the means to determine the few days during each menstrual cycle when they are fertile and another method of birth control is needed.

Although to date there are FAM studies in progress, none have completely documented the effectiveness of the use of barrier and spermicidal methods of contraception during the fertile time. Many family planning professionals believe that the effectiveness rates should be about the same as the rates achieved when the diaphragm, condom, and spermicide are used throughout the menstrual cycle.

Because FAM uses these other methods only during the fertile time, people may actually use them more conscientiously and correctly, resulting in fewer unplanned pregnancies.

The reasons people choose to use natural family planning or fertility awareness methods are certainly varied and complex. To some, NFP is a way of life. It is not only a method of birth control, but a total way that a woman and man relate to each other, spiritually, emotionally, and physically. NFP is also a method that is compatible with the teachings of certain religions. For others, NFP is used because it is in keeping with their beliefs about their health. Some people desire to eliminate as many chemicals as possible from their lifestyle. And for some, natural family planning is the only method of birth control they can or want to use, due to prior physical and/or emotional problems with other methods of birth control. The numbers of people using the fertility awareness method appear to be growing because it seems that they wish to use the natural language of the body in combination with a method of birth control they are comfortable with. In the end, the method chosen will depend upon a number of factors including the physical, emotional, sexual, and spiritual needs of the person.

Now that we've briefly introduced natural family planning and fertility awareness methods to you, and given you an idea of how poorly reproduction was understood in the past, it's time to begin learning how well reproduction and these new methods of natural family planning are understood today.

Chapter 3

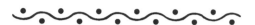

All the Parts "Down There" and How They Work—The Man

Men's and women's reproductive systems have similarities and obvious differences, and each goes through its own special and wondrous patterns to allow pregnancy to occur—at least some of the time.

Learning how these patterns and systems work and using the knowledge of fertility signs allow a couple to make certain choices about their lovemaking.

Located at the base of the brain is a small gland called the **pituitary gland**. Basically, it controls the reproductive system by sending hormonal signals in both men and women. (**Hormones** are chemicals that take messages from glands to other parts of the body, causing them to perform special and specific tasks.)

The pituitary gland begins to work more actively around the time a boy reaches the age of 8–12. As a result, a time of physical and emotional change known as **puberty** begins, which lasts about 4 years. During these years the major male hormone, **testosterone,** plays an important part in the development of the boy's body. For example, testosterone causes the growth of body hair and sex organs, including the penis. Sexual feelings also begin to increase under the influence of testosterone. This is the time a boy begins to experience "wet dreams," known as nocturnal emissions—a normal involuntary ejaculation which occurs when the boy is asleep. (Ejaculation is the release of semen from the penis.)

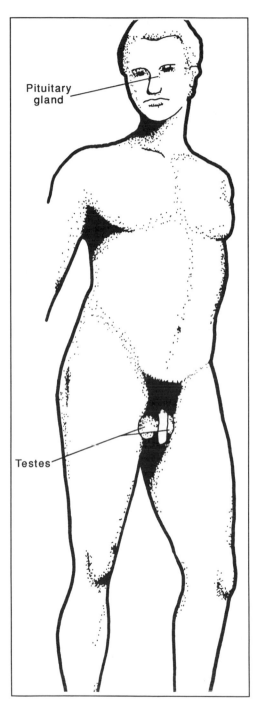

Figure 1 Pituitary Gland and Testes

During puberty, the pituitary gland sends a message to the **testes,** the male sex glands.

As a result of this message, the testes begin to produce sperm and testosterone. The testes are a pair of oval-shaped organs that produce about 50,000,000 sperm each day. They are protected by two sacs of loose, thin tissue known as the **scrotum.** The scrotum and testes are located on the outside of the man's body for a very specific reason—their anatomical positioning keeps them cooler than normal body temperature, and cool temperature is needed for sperm production. Once sperm are produced in the testes, they travel to the **epididymis,** an area where they become fully developed. This is where they will wait until they begin their journey through the rest of the man's reproductive system.

Shortly before ejaculation, the sperm leave the epididymis and move along the **vas deferens,** a pair of 20-inch-long tubes that carry sperm to the **seminal vesicles.** These sac-like structures produce seminal fluid that mixes with the sperm. Sperm and seminal fluid continue traveling through the vas deferens, which goes around the side of the bladder, to the **prostate gland.** This gland is the size and shape of an acorn and produces a thin, milky fluid which also nourishes the sperm. When sperm mixes with fluid from the seminal vesicles and prostate gland, semen is formed, which moves into the pas-

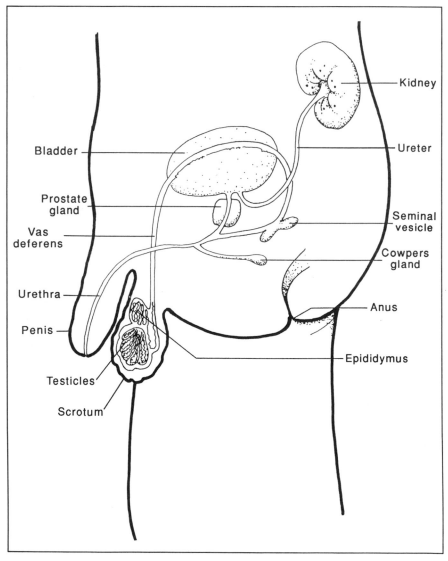

Figure 2 Male Reproductive System

sageway of the **ejaculatory duct.** By the time sperm travel and fluid production begins, the man's penis has become swollen. The swelling is caused by an increase in the amount of blood flowing into the tissues of the penis. The tube that runs through the center of the penis is called the **urethra.** Usually the urethra serves as the exit for urine from the man's body, but during ejaculation the urethra serves as an exit for the semen. A pair of sac-like glands known as the **Cowpers glands** produce a fluid that also helps sperm live. When a man is sexually aroused and before he ejaculates, the fluid travels through the urethra to the tip of the penis.

Some researchers feel that these drops of fluid from the Cowpers glands contain enough sperm to cause a pregnancy. This means that if the tip of the penis touches the outside of the vagina during a woman's fertile time, pregnancy may occur. When the penis touches the vagina, it is called "genital to genital contact." As we will discuss later, *no genital to genital contact* should occur during the woman's fertile days if the couple wishes to avoid a pregnancy. When ejaculation is about to occur, muscles in the reproductive system begin to contract or move to push the semen through the urethra to the outside of the man's body.

Two important facts to remember:

1. The man is fertile every day from puberty until about the age of 70

2. Pregnancy may occur if even just the tip of the penis touches the outside of the vagina during the woman's fertile days

Chapter 4

All the Parts "Down There" and How They Work—The Woman

The woman's fertility pattern is quite different from the man's. While the man is fertile every day, the woman is fertile approximately 5–7 days during each menstrual cycle. To understand why this is so is to learn how the woman's reproductive system works. This can be done by first looking at the part of the system located on the outside of the woman's body. This part is called the external genitalia, or outer reproductive organs.

At the top of these is the **mons veneris** (named after Venus, the goddess of love). It is a pad of fatty tissue that covers the pubic bone and at puberty becomes covered with pubic hair. The mons veneris helps to protect the internal reproductive organs. Below it is the **vaginal opening** or the entrance to the **vaginal canal.** This opening allows for the final exit of menstrual blood from the body. The vaginal canal widens to allow for intercourse and also expands to aid in the birth of a baby. Often, at birth, a baby girl has a paper-thin tissue that partially and sometimes totally covers the vaginal opening. This tissue, known as the **hymen,** can easily be stretched by insertion of a tampon, finger, or penis. Once this stretching occurs, irregular-looking pieces of the hymen are left around the vaginal opening. These pieces are known as the **hymenal tags.**

Located on either side of the vaginal opening are two sets of vaginal lips. The outer set is made of fatty tissue covered with skin that contains oil-producing glands. These outer lips are covered, to some degree, with pubic hair. The inner set of lips are hairless and do not contain oil-producing glands. This set is made of folds of soft skin. Together, the **labia majora** (outer lips) and **labia minora** (inner lips) protect the vaginal opening when a woman is not sexually aroused. When a woman does become sexually aroused, blood flows into the vaginal lips, causing them to fill with blood and flatten out away from the vagina—allowing for the insertion of the penis. The **clitoris,** a small organ located below the mons veneris and above the vaginal opening, is made of the same kind of tissue as the penis. The clitoris becomes filled with blood during sexual arousal, causing it to become firm and erect. It contains many nerve endings which make it the main area of sexual arousal for many women. The clitoris is protected by a covering called the **hood,** which is formed by the joining of the inner lips above the clitoris.

Below the clitoris and above the vaginal entrance is the urinary opening, called the **urethral meatus.** This opening is the entrance to the urethra, a tube leading to the bladder. The urinary opening serves as the passageway for the urine to travel from the bladder to the outside of the body. Below the vaginal opening is the **perineum.** This area of tissue is often cut during the birth of a baby to allow the baby easier passage out of the vaginal opening. The perineum also separates the vaginal opening from the **anus,** the muscular opening of the **rectum** that serves as the exit for the body's solid waste materials.

The **vulva** is the name given to all of the external genitalia that we've just described. Women often wonder if their vulva looks normal. The amount of pubic hair, size of the vaginal lips, and clitoris form a unique "style" for each woman. If a woman places a mirror between her thighs, she can see her external organs. The woman comfortable doing this can become better acquainted with her body. She can learn what is normal for her. In other words, a woman who takes the time to look and touch these various parts of her body can learn to feel comfortable with her own body and gain a fuller understanding and awareness of it. This may help her overcome any uncomfortable feelings she may have about the outside of her reproductive system.

As we have mentioned, many of the external parts of the woman's reproductive system help to protect the internal reproductive organs. The internal reproductive organs work together to enable a woman to become pregnant and nourish the pregnancy through nine months of development.

Beginning with the **uterus,** we see a hollow, muscular organ that is somewhat pear-shaped. It is only about 3 inches long and provides the space for the fetus to be nourished during the nine months of development. The innermost lining of the uterus is

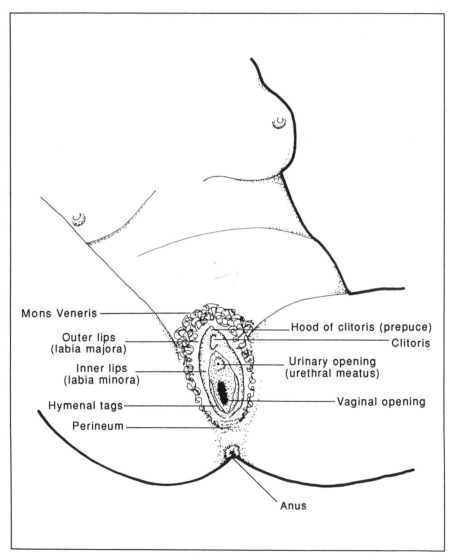

Figure 3 External Female Reproductive Anatomy

called the **endometrium.** This lining becomes rich in blood supply and nutrients necessary for a pregnancy to occur and develop.

If the woman doesn't become pregnant during her cycle, the lining breaks down, causing bleeding. This is called **menstruation.** The menstrual blood leaves the uterus through its bottom opening, known as the **cervix.** The cervix is often referred to as the neck of the uterus because it looks like a small neck sticking out at the very top of the vagina. The cervix has an opening that allows the sperm to enter the uterus during the fertile days of the menstrual cycle. The cervix also has glands made up of special cells that produce a fluid called **cervical mucus.** During the fertile days of the menstrual cycle this mucus has a special consistency and is made of certain substances that allow sperm to live and travel through the woman's reproductive system to enable pregnancy to occur.

A 4–6-inch elastic, muscular tube is the connection between the vaginal opening and the cervix. Commonly called the birth canal or vaginal canal, this tube has the ability to expand during sexual arousal, allowing sexual intercourse. It also expands to allow the birth of a baby. When a woman is sexually aroused the blood vessels in the lining of the vaginal canal become full, causing a slippery liquid to be produced. This liquid lubricates the vaginal canal, enabling a woman to have comfortable intercourse.

Vaginal and uterine muscles, as well as muscles around the reproductive organs, contract if a woman experiences an orgasm. (See the Bibliography for references if you want more detailed information about the changes in men's and women's bodies during lovemaking and orgasm.)

Two very small primary sex organs, known as the **ovaries,** are located on each side of the uterus. At birth, a baby girl has all of the immature eggs (called **ova**) in her ovaries that she will ever need. At birth there are about two million of them, and each is surrounded by a capsule called the **follicle.** The human egg can be compared to the chicken egg in a general way. The center of the chicken egg has a yolk surrounded by a white fluid and a shell to protect the whole egg. The human egg, smaller than a grain of sand, forms the center and has fluid around it. This entire structure is called the follicle. At some point during each menstrual cycle an egg will fully develop and be released from its follicle and ovary. The egg is then picked up by one of the **fallopian tubes**. The fallopian tubes are a pair of narrow, muscular passageways. They are thin, about 4 inches in length, and have finger-like ends called **fimbriae.** The fimbriae encircle the ovary and pick up the egg. The outer portion of the tube is where the egg will wait for about 24 hours. If sperm have not traveled through the uterus and up the fallopian tube before the time the egg has arrived, or within the next 24 hours, the egg will not be fertilized. Eventually, it will be absorbed in the reproductive system and usually does not leave the body in the menstrual blood. If the egg is fertilized, it will begin

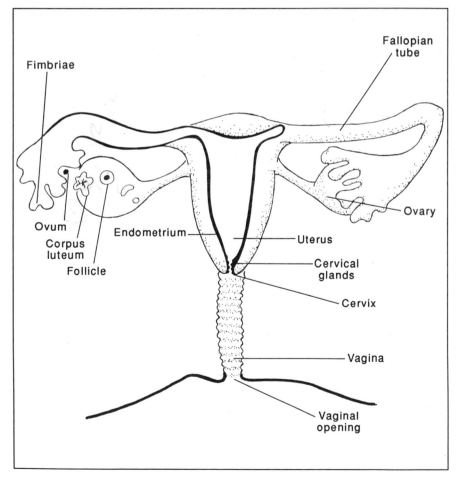

Figure 4 Female Internal Reproductive Organs

a journey of approximately one week down the fallopian tube, into the uterus, and burrow itself into the rich lining of the uterus, which has been preparing for the possibility of pregnancy. This is called **implantation.** The uterine lining is a perfect home for the fertilized egg, allowing it to develop into a baby within nine months.

For most young girls puberty begins between the ages of 8 and 13. As with the boy, the process lasts about four years, allowing for physical and sexual maturity to take place. Generally, the first sign of puberty is breast development, followed by growth of underarm and pubic hair. One of the last events of puberty is the start of menstrual bleeding. Although the beginning of menstrual bleeding means the ovaries have reached an adult level of development, the release of the first egg may not begin for 1–2 years after this first menstrual period. Once the eggs begin to be released, the young girl is fertile and can become pregnant.

Usually one egg leaves the ovary during each fertility cycle. By the time a woman reaches menopause, about 400 will have been released.

Ovulation, or the release of the egg from the ovary, is the MAIN EVENT of the fertility cycle. The fertility cycle, commonly known as the **menstrual cycle,** spans many days. Although a menstrual cycle can be somewhat shorter or longer, it usually ranges from 24–35 days in length. It is not unusual for a woman's menstrual cycle to vary from 2–7 days in length from month to month. For example, the same woman may have cycles that are 25 days long, 27 days

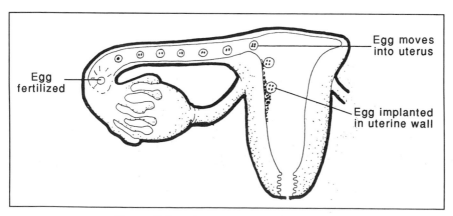

Figure 5 Fertilization and Implantation

long, and still other cycles 32 days long. And that is okay—it is normal for her. It is also normal for the number of days and amount of bleeding to change with different menstrual cycles.

A menstrual cycle always begins the first day any sign of menstrual bleeding appears and ends the day before menstrual bleeding begins again. For example, let's say Mary's menstrual bleeding began April 1. Her next menstrual bleeding began April 30. Therefore, her menstrual cycle during April was 29 days long. About the time menstrual bleeding begins, the **pituitary gland** sends messages to the ovaries signaling them to continue their growth of several eggs. As the follicles and eggs are maturing, the follicles surrounding the eggs also start to produce one of the major female hormones, **estrogen.** The hormone estrogen is responsible for causing the young girl's body to develop into the body of a woman. Estrogen also causes the lining of the uterus to grow and develop the proper blood supply and nutrients necessary for implantation (attachment) of the fertilized egg to the lining of the uterus. A woman cannot feel this change. However, other changes caused by estrogen can be seen and felt; one is cervical mucus. **Fertile cervical mucus** is produced as the amount of estrogen increases. Fertile mucus has certain qualities that will enable sperm to stay healthy and able to fertilize an egg from 3 and perhaps even up to 5 days! That means a woman can have intercourse on Monday and, if fertile mucus is present, the sperm can be waiting in the reproductive system to fertilize an egg—even if it isn't released from the ovary until Friday! *The fact that sperm may be able to fertilize the egg up to 5 days after intercourse is important to remember for the successful use of natural family planning.*

This cervical mucus may also help filter out unhealthy sperm. It contains channels that form "super-

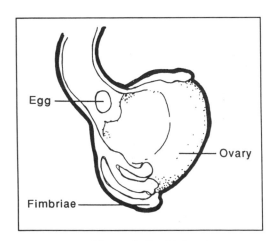

Figure 6 Ovulation

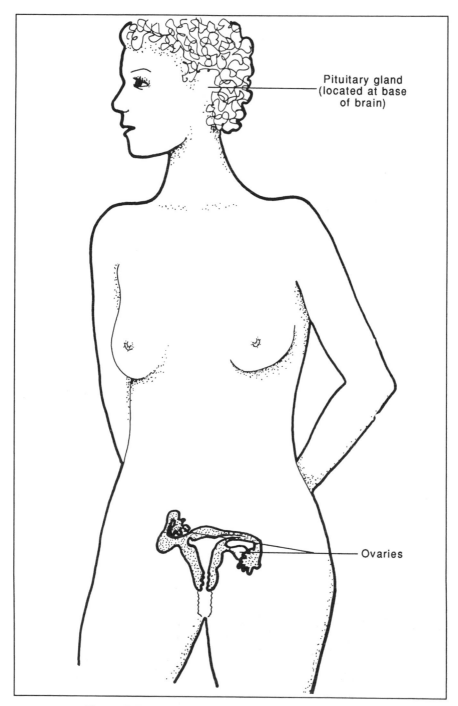

Pituitary gland
(located at base
of brain)

Ovaries

Figure 7 Pituitary Gland and Reproductive Organs

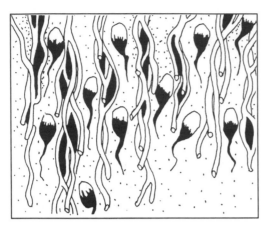

Figure 8 Fertile Mucus

highways" that vibrate, helping to push the sperm up into the uterus.

Estrogen also produces a change in the position of the uterus, causing the cervix to move upward in the vaginal canal. Estrogen also causes the cervix to soften and its opening to widen. All of these changes help sperm to travel easily into the uterus. The changes in both the mucus and the cervix can be observed by the woman, enabling her to determine her days of fertility. *Cervical mucus and changes in the cervix are two main fertility signs used to achieve or prevent a pregnancy.*

Once the eggs have reached a certain level of maturity and estrogen is at a proper level in the woman's body, the pituitary gland sends another message to the ovary signaling one of the eggs to complete its development and leave the ovary. (The remaining several eggs that were also growing stop developing and will never grow again.) The egg leaves its follicle and enters the fallopian tube. The follicle then turns into an entirely different structure that is yellow in color. This is the **corpus luteum** (Latin for "yellow body"). The corpus luteum produces large amounts of **progesterone**—the second major female hormone. Once ovulation has taken place, progesterone controls the remainder of the menstrual cycle. One of its jobs is to change the lining of the uterus so that within 5–7 days after the egg has been released, the uterine lining is com-

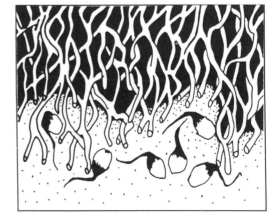

Figure 9 Infertile Mucus

pletely prepared to receive a fertilized egg. A large amount of progesterone helps stop the ovaries from releasing more eggs, meaning once ovulation occurs, it will not happen again later in that same menstrual cycle. Occasionally a second (and, rarely, a third or fourth) egg will be released, but if that happens, it will be within 24 hours after the release of the first egg. This explains the reason for non-identical, fraternal twins. About 1% of all babies born in the U.S. are non-identical twins.

After one or perhaps two eggs are released, no more will be released during the cycle. Since there are no more eggs released, there is no further chance of pregnancy. This is another important factor to remember in using fertility signs to prevent pregnancy.

Progesterone also causes the production of **infertile cervical mucus**. After ovulation the mucus produced destroys sperm and blocks it from traveling into the uterus. The cervix lowers in the vaginal canal and becomes firm, and the opening closes. These natural occurrences prevent sperm or any other foreign matter from entering the uterus and harming a pregnancy should one have occurred. Once again, these special changes in the mucus and cervix can enable a woman to identify the days when she is infertile, or unable to become pregnant.

In addition to changes in mucus and the cervix, changes in basal body temperature provide an invaluable sign to help a woman determine when she is no longer fertile. Shortly before, during, or shortly after ovulation, the body temperature rises from about three-tenths of a degree to one full degree Fahrenheit (0.3°–1.0°F) higher than it had been up to that point. This happens because progesterone is a heat-producing hormone. Once the temperature has risen, it will remain high for 12–16 days, or until the next menstrual cycle begins. This is because the corpus luteum produces progesterone for several days, keeping the uterine lining prepared for the possibility of pregnancy. If pregnancy doesn't occur, the corpus luteum stops working and the hormone levels decrease. Thus, the hormones are no longer present in the quantity needed to keep the uterine lining in place. The lining breaks down, accompanied by bleeding. This is the menstrual flow, which begins a new menstrual cycle. Menstrual cycles continue until the ovaries have "run out" of eggs. This takes place about the age of

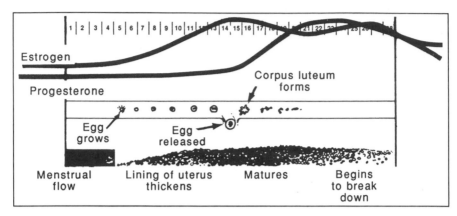

Figure 10 Menstrual Cycle

50. Once bleeding has ceased for one full year, a woman has reached menopause, and she can no longer become pregnant.

Menstrual bleeding is called **menses** from the Latin word for "monthly." It is more commonly referred to by a variety of names and phrases such as: "period," "friend," "curse," "falling off the roof," and "being on the rag." Throughout history and even today, menstrual bleeding has been thought of more often as a "curse" than a "friend"! There are many reasons for this. During ancient times, bleeding was associated with the life process. This meant that life went on as long as the blood stayed in the body. To bleed meant to be injured and frequently to die. Therefore, for a woman to bleed and not be hurt was an unexplained mystery. Almost every religion and culture has written about this mystery of women, and often in a negative way. It was felt that women were possessed either by evil or by good spirits. For a period of time women were considered to be goddesses. They were felt to possess supernatural powers. If women could control the life force, they could also control the weather, the growth of crops, birth, and death.

This powerful, godlike role given to women soon turned into a role very much the opposite. As soon as the early civilizations realized women who continued menstruating were not helping to increase the population, menstruation became a "curse." Women were said to be possessed by the devil and were called witches. When they were menstruating, they were considered to be dangerous to men. In fact, women were blamed for just about everything. If crops died, milk curdled, meat spoiled, or a tornado or hurricane came along, guess who was blamed? In some areas of the world, women had to live in special places away from their homes during menstruation. This was to protect everyone from harm, since the look from a menstruating woman was said to soften men's bones and prevent them from fighting well during a battle.

Obviously this attitude about menstruation was based upon ignorance and carried too far. Many women today still feel the effects of this history. Many women and men feel that menstruation is unclean, instead of viewing it as the end of one fertility cycle and the beginning of the next. Nothing more, nothing less.

TO REVIEW

During the first part of the menstrual cycle, the eggs develop and the cervix rises, softens, opens and produces fertile mucus. These changes let sperm live and travel to the egg. They can also help a woman identify the time when she can become pregnant, called fertile days.

Once the egg leaves its follicle, the cervix closes and infertile mucus is produced. These changes help to protect a pregnancy if it should occur. The basal body temperature also rises. All of these changes help a woman identify the time when she cannot become pregnant, called infertile days.

YOUR NOTES:

_____

_____

_____

_____

_____

_____

_____

Chapter 5

Primary Fertility Signs:
The Three Major Ones

In the spring, a good gardener knows the signs for the time to plant. The pattern of the seasons is nature's language to the gardener. Nature's language to the woman is fertility signs.

It's important to learn all you can about your fertility cycle so that you are able to use your method of family planning as effectively as possible. *Awareness is important.* In this section we emphasize a special kind of awareness—*fertility awareness:* learning about fertility signs and their patterns.

The three most important fertility signs are:

- cervical mucus changes

- basal body temperature changes

- cervical changes

CERVICAL MUCUS CHANGES

Cervical mucus is a substance that every woman produces naturally. It is one of the three most important fertility signs your body offers you, and can be thought of as a special signal from your body telling you about your reproductive system. It tells you when you are able to become pregnant, as well as when you are not able to become pregnant. Cervical mucus is normal, it is healthy, it is important, and it can be easy to learn and understand.

This mucus is produced by very small glands in the cervix and it changes in ways that you can see and feel throughout your menstrual cycle. During certain days of the menstrual cycle, the mucus will be of either the fertile or infertile type. Fertile mucus is present a few days before and during the time of ovulation. Infertile mucus is present at other times of the menstrual cycle when pregnancy cannot occur.

Remember: Fertile mucus helps a woman become pregnant; infertile mucus helps a woman prevent pregnancy.

Both fertile and infertile mucus have their own special
— color
— amount
— feel
and you can learn to identify each kind.

After the menstrual flow ends, one of three changes will occur in the mucus pattern.

Change Number 1. You may not have any mucus for one day or more. Days without any mucus are called "dry days." In fact, your vaginal area around the vaginal opening and lips may "feel" dry. Some women notice this dryness toward the end of their menstrual flow because, in removing a tampon, they experience discomfort. Dryness may also be felt during love-making. You may not experience the same amount of vaginal wetness while making love on these dry days as you experience at other times in your menstrual cycle.

Change Number 2. When the menstrual flow ends, you may produce a mucus that is sticky, pasty, or crumbly. It sometimes resembles old-fashioned library paste, looking whitish-yellow on your underwear. (Figure 11) It is not a wet-feeling mucus. Since it has very little moisture, it causes the vaginal area to feel dry or sticky.

Change Number 3. When the menstrual flow ends, you may produce a wet-feeling mucus that appears creamy and white. (Figure 12) This type of mucus may create a wet feeling around the vaginal opening.

To sum up, once the menstrual flow ends, you may experience:

1. A dry feeling at the opening of the vagina, with no mucus present

2. A dry or sticky feeling at the opening of the vagina, with sticky, pasty, crumbly mucus

3. A wet feeling at the opening of the vagina with a wet-feeling mucus

Regardless of whether you are dry or you begin to produce non-wet or wet mucus after the menstrual flow ends, the closer the approach of ovulation, the wetter the mucus becomes. This is due to the fact that in the beginning of the menstrual cycle your body's estrogen level is low. As ovulation approaches, the increase of estrogen causes glands in the cervix to produce the wetter mucus.

In addition, the amount of mucus can increase, and it usually becomes clearer in color. It may even be pink, tinged with blood, and can be stretched between two fingers. (Figure 13) This type of mucus has the appearance and texture of raw egg-white. Known as **spinnbarkeit** (pronounced spin-bar-kite), it can look like the shimmering strands of a spider web. It is likely that you will notice a wet feeling at the opening of your vagina along with an increase of wet mucus on your underwear. Some women have misunderstood this wet mucus, considering it to be the sign of a vaginal infection. This is not so!

During the time when your mucus is the wet-

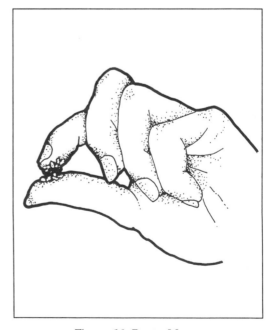

Figure 11 Pasty Mucus

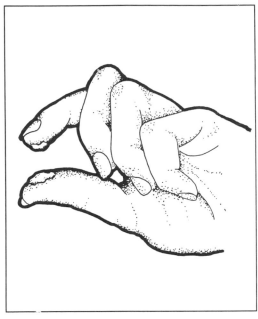

Figure 12 Creamy Mucus

test and most slippery, your estrogen level is at its highest. This sign allows you to know that ovulation has recently taken place or will occur within a few days.

Soon after ovulation, the progesterone level begins to rise in your body, causing other changes in the cervical mucus. As it rises, the wet feeling at the outside of your vaginal opening disappears, and the mucus becomes sticky, pasty, and dry. Some women have a constant dry feeling at the outside of the vagina because they do not have any mucus for the remainder of their menstrual cycle. Other women continue to have pasty mucus and dry vaginal feelings until their next menstrual cycle begins. A few days prior to menstrual bleeding some women notice a wet discharge and wet feeling at the outside of the vaginal opening. Although the mucus feels wet, it is not fertile mucus. It is fluid from the lining of the uterus that flows out of the vagina prior to the start of menstrual bleeding.

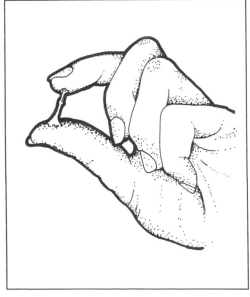

Figure 13 Stretchy Mucus

Many women notice these normal mucus changes throughout their menstrual cycles—the wet and dry feelings, the increase and decrease in vaginal secretions, and the color changes—yet have never associated these changes with their fertility patterns.

Cervical mucus changes and vaginal feelings (or sensations) are the main fertility signs, which give advance notice that ovulation is going to happen.

Is it correct to say that ovulation took place on the day of the greatest amount of stretchy, wet mucus? *No!* This type of mucus simply tells you that the time of ovulation is close.

We know that when menstrual bleeding ends, the appearance of any mucus, whether it feels wet or not, means an egg has begun growing and may soon be released.

WARNING! The change from the sticky, pasty, crumbly infertile type of mucus to the wet, fertile type of mucus can be difficult to see and feel when you are first learning about your mucus changes. Therefore, you may miss detecting a small amount of fertile mucus mixed with infertile mucus. In addition, some women may see this infertile mucus, but slippery, stretchy, and wet fertile mucus can be up in the cervix. It can take a day or so for this mucus to travel to the vaginal opening where it can be seen. Therefore, after the menstrual bleeding ends, *any type of mucus that appears before ovulation is considered fertile.*

This means that if intercourse takes place when *any* type of mucus is seen before ovulation, a pregnancy may result.

BASAL BODY TEMPERATURE

The second primary fertility sign is your basal body temperature. This is the temperature of your body at rest. When it is taken daily, you will see it rise and fall in a definite pattern that can be used to help you determine when your infertile days begin after ovulation.

When the menstrual flow starts, your temperature may still be high from the progesterone produced during the previous menstrual cycle. If it is, your basal body temperature will usually drop down to a low level by the time the menstrual flow ends, and will remain low until around the time of ovulation. This low level usually ranges from 96°–97.4° Fahrenheit (F) or 35.4°–36.8° Centigrade (C), although for some women it can be somewhat higher. Shortly before, during, or after ovulation, it will rise to a higher level, usually from 0.3°–1.0°F (0.15°–0.5°C) higher than the previous low temperatures.

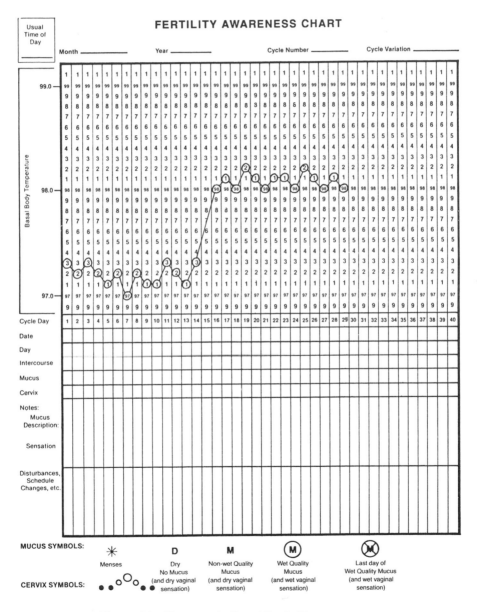

Figure 14 Changes in Basal Body Temperature

Basal body temperature will remain high for about 12–16 days. Menstrual bleeding usually occurs when the temperature begins to fall. If your basal body temperature remains high longer than 20 days and sexual intercourse occurred during a fertile time, this can be a reliable sign of pregnancy.

Is it correct to say that ovulation takes place the day before the temperature rise? NO! It often does, but it can also take place the day of the temperature rise, the day after the rise, and even a few days before the rise. Yet once the temperature goes up and stays high for 3 days, it is proof that the egg has been released.

CHANGES IN THE CERVIX

The third primary fertility sign is changes in the cervix. Although cervical changes do not have to be observed to determine days of fertility and infertility, they can provide additional information about a woman's fertility pattern.

During the menstrual period, the cervix is usually easy to touch with a finger. The area surrounding its opening is soft and widened to allow for the menstrual flow.

When the period ends, the cervix is still usually easy to feel. If you touch it with your finger, you can feel that your cervix is closer to your vaginal opening and it feels firm, like the tip of a nose or a small rubber ball, and the opening is closed.

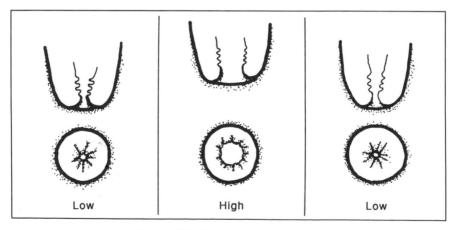

Figure 15 Changes in the Cervix

In a woman who has not had a vaginal delivery, the opening is like a dimple, whereas the woman who has delivered vaginally may have a cervical opening that feels irregular and wide. Also, if you have delivered children vaginally you may have relaxed support of the uterus, making it difficult to feel the rising and lowering of the cervix.

As ovulation approaches, the rising estrogen levels cause the cervix to move away from the vaginal opening. Therefore, you will have to insert a finger further into the vagina to feel it. Also, the cervical opening begins to widen and the area surrounding it softens, so that the texture of the area around the cervical opening can be compared to the softness of the lips. This rising and opening of the cervix occur to help sperm travel into the uterus.

After ovulation, the rising progesterone level causes the cervix once again to lower in the vaginal canal and be easier to reach. It becomes firmer, and the cervical opening becomes smaller. These changes help prevent sperm from entering the uterus.

Is it correct to say that ovulation took place when the cervix was at its highest, most soft and open time? NO! The cervix signals you that the egg is preparing to leave the ovary. Cervical changes cannot tell you the exact day ovulation takes place.

Just as some women have noticed their normally changing mucus signs without connecting them to their fertility patterns, some are familiar with their cervical changes. For example, inserting a tampon or having intercourse in certain positions can be uncomfortable when the cervix is in its low position.

TO REVIEW:

The main fertility signs are

- cervical mucus and vaginal feelings

- basal body temperature

- changes in the cervix

These enable you to make accurate and sensible choices concerning your fertility. The fertility signs—cannot be used to determine the exact day of ovulation. Instead, they are used to identify the fertile and infertile days of each menstrual cycle. Since you are able to do this, you will have information that can lead to an excellent way of planning sexual intercourse to either achieve or prevent pregnancy.

YOUR NOTES:

_____

_____

_____

_____

_____

_____

_____

_____

_____

Chapter 6

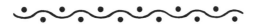

Secondary Fertility Signs

You have naturally occurring signs that will enable you to know when the egg is about to be released, as well as when it has been released, and when it can no longer be fertilized. Though you won't be able to know the exact time and day of ovulation, by observing your fertility signs you can accurately determine the days when you can or cannot become pregnant.

Remember, you have three primary fertility signs:

1. Cervical mucus can be used to determine when the fertile days begin and end. It serves as a sign of approaching ovulation and can also be used to know when ovulation has taken place

2. Basal body temperature can be used to know when ovulation has taken place and the fertile days have ended

3. Cervical changes can provide you with additional information about the approach and end of the fertile days

Also, remember these facts:

- the first day of the menstrual cycle begins with the first day of bleeding

- the cycle ends the day before the next bleeding begins

- the menstrual cycle is your fertility cycle

- ovulation occurs about 12–16 days before menstrual bleeding

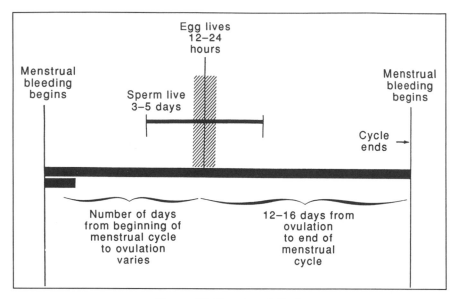

Figure 16 Menstrual Cycle

- ovulation can take place a few to several days after a menstrual cycle begins

- an egg is able to be fertilized for about 24 hours after ovulation

- sperm may be capable of fertilizing the egg up to 5 days when fertile cervical mucus is present

- the primary fertility signs reflect all this information

These facts make up the major principles for the use of fertility signs to prevent or achieve a pregnancy.

Other changes that may occur in a woman's body around the time of ovulation provide additional information about her own unique fertility pattern. These are called secondary fertility signs, and are useful to learn. But since not all women experience them, they are not as dependable for determining the fertile and infertile times as cervical mucus and basal body temperature.

As ovulation approaches, the body's oil-producing glands secrete less oil. This causes a decrease in oily skin and, for some women, a clearer complexion. Some women also find their bodies

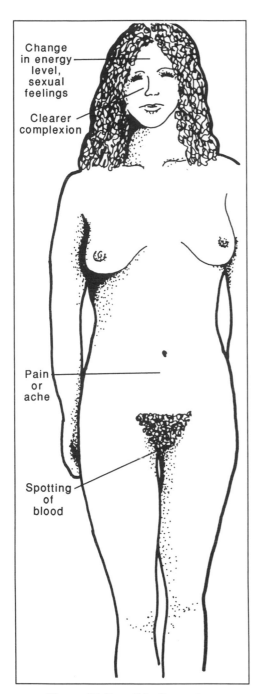

Change in energy level, sexual feelings

Clearer complexion

Pain or ache

Spotting of blood

Figure 17 Possible Secondary Fertility Signs as Ovulation Nears

begin to "hold water," called fluid retention. Fluid retention causes a slight bloated feeling, slight breast tenderness, and even irritability. These feelings are not as severe as those experienced premenstrually and usually last for only a day or two.

Some women notice an increase in energy during the days leading up to ovulation. In fact, some women even experience a sharper sense of vision, smell, and taste as ovulation approaches.

A dull ache or pain may occur in the pelvic area shortly before, during, or shortly after ovulation. This pain or ache may last a few minutes or a few days. It may occur on one side of the pelvic area or on both sides. It may travel down one or both legs and even around to the lower back. This pain may be accompanied by spotting or a light flow of blood.

Around the time of ovulation, some women notice an increase in sexual feelings. Others experience no change or even a decrease in sexual feelings.

Some women experience all of these changes while others experience only a few. For those women who experience them, these changes can give additional information about their own special fertility patterns.

As menstruation nears, the body's oil-producing glands secrete more oil, causing an increase in acne and oily skin. Cramping, leg aches, and backaches can occur. Your body may hold more fluid, causing breast tenderness. You may also experience itching of the nipples, headaches, and mood changes. Some women notice an increase or decrease in sexual feelings at this time.

There are over 100 premenstrual symptoms, collectively known as premenstrual syndrome, which can negatively affect a woman's life up to several days before her menstrual bleeding begins. (See the Bibliography for books that discuss premenstrual symptoms in detail as well as various ways to treat them.)

There are different theories about the causes and treatment of premenstrual syndrome. Some people feel that the use of progesterone is the answer. Others believe that treatment should include the use of specific vitamins combined with special diets, exercises, and stress-reduction techniques. If you find that you, or someone you know, is experiencing certain physical and/or emotional changes 1–14 days before menstruation, you should know that help is available. You can read information about premenstrual syndrome and discuss it with your physician, as well as contact organizations that have been formed to help women with this problem.

A WORD ABOUT PRIMARY
AND SECONDARY FERTILITY SIGNS

Fertility signs cannot be used to determine the exact day of ovulation. However, when fertility signs are observed carefully, you can learn the approximate time of ovulation and, most importantly, you can tell when the time of ovulation is approaching as well as when it has occurred. Therefore, you will see and feel the beginning of your fertile time early enough in the menstrual cycle to prevent or achieve a pregnancy. You will also know when your fertile time has ended.

TO REVIEW

During the fertility cycle you can experience various fertility signs
—three primary and several secondary ones.

Primary Signs

- Cervical mucus and vaginal feelings

- Basal body temperature

- Cervical changes

Possible Secondary Signs

- Clearing of complexion

- Decrease in hair and body oil production

- Water retention

- Aches or pain in lower body

- Increased sensitivity in skin and breasts

- Increased energy level

- Increased or decreased sexual feelings

It is important for you to keep a record of as many bodily
changes as possible. By keeping a chart of your individual pattern
of fertility signs, you will be able to gain a clearer understanding of
the fertile and infertile times of your menstrual cycle. It will also
increase your awareness of your own normal bodily changes.

YOUR NOTES:

_____

_____

_____

_____

_____

Chapter 7

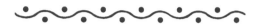

Observing the Way to Awareness

The first step in learning about your own fertility pattern is to observe it carefully. To accomplish this, we recommend that you use as many fertility signs as you are comfortable with to prevent pregnancy. Since you will be establishing a new habit, learning accurate information, and developing your fertility awareness, it is important that you check your fertility signs every day until you feel you have learned your fertility pattern well.

You need only 10–15 minutes each day to observe fertility signs accurately. As you gain experience, you will get better and better, decreasing the time spent. In fact, once you learn your own fertility cycle and enter the infertile part of your menstrual cycle after ovulation, it is not necessary to check your signs for the remainder of that cycle.

Checking your fertility signs can be compared to the daily habit of brushing your teeth. It can be done automatically and regularly, and takes a few minutes. You pick up the toothbrush, squeeze the tube of toothpaste and brush your teeth—without thinking. Placing a thermometer under your tongue and/or looking at cervical mucus and other signs can also become part of your daily routine. Before long it's habit, and you do it without giving it a second thought.

CERVICAL MUCUS OBSERVATION

When you wake up in the morning, you should find out about your cervical mucus and vaginal sensations before you bathe and wash them away. Ask yourself this question: "Does the area at the outside of the vaginal opening and in the vaginal opening feel wet or dry?" Vaginal sensations, or what you feel on the outside of your vagina (by thinking about it), depend on whether mucus is present and on the quality of this mucus. For example, wet mucus will make the outside of the vagina feel wet. And sticky, pasty, and crumbly mucus that does not feel significantly wet will make the outside of the vagina feel dry. An absence of mucus also causes the outside of the vagina to feel dry.

Vaginal sensations are also called vaginal feelings. They are not experienced by touching the vaginal area with the fingers. They are feelings a woman mentally "tunes into." While walking, sitting, and lying down, a woman needs to ask herself, "Do I feel wet or dry?" Through continuous practice, assessing vaginal sensations becomes easier and easier. In fact, some women become so experienced with evaluating their vaginal sensations they know which type of mucus they are producing without even using the external mucus checking technique. Even if this level of experience is gained, we still strongly suggest that the woman continue with regular mucus checking. Combining knowledge of vaginal sensations and cervical mucus is the ideal way to go when using this knowledge to prevent pregnancy.

Once you have decided how the outside of the vagina feels, the next step is external checking. This technique enables you to see if mucus is present, as well as to assess its quality, color, and amount.

There are three steps to external checking:

1. Take a piece of folded white toilet tissue and wipe the outside of the vaginal opening

2. Next, look at the toilet tissue and answer these questions:
   — Is there any mucus on the toilet tissue?
   — If so, what color is it?
   — How much mucus is on the toilet tissue?

3. Then check how the mucus feels
   — Take a sample of the mucus between two fingers to determine how it feels

— Open the fingers slowly apart to see if the mucus stretches or just forms little peaks
— Does the mucus feel sticky, pasty and crumbly or does it feel wet? Does it feel stretchy and slippery?
— *Your cervical mucus should be checked several times during the day because mucus can change during the day.* For example, it can be pasty and sticky in the morning and afternoon, but by nighttime it can be wet and stretchy. The more often you check your mucus, the better. Many women find it convenient to check their cervical mucus each time they go to the bathroom

TO REVIEW

Vaginal Sensations

• How does the outside of the vaginal area feel?

— Is it wet feeling?

— Is it dry feeling?

Cervical Mucus

• Collect some mucus and look at it

— Is it clear or cloudy?

— Is it creamy?

• Feel the mucus

— Is it slippery?

— Is it pasty?

— Is it crumbly?

— Try to stretch the mucus between your fingers

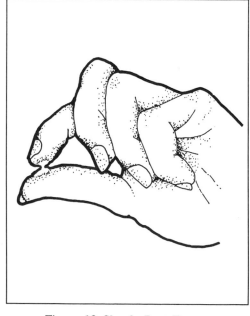

Figure 18 Slowly Part Fingers

KEGEL EXERCISE

No doubt you have had to go to the bathroom when there was no bathroom in sight. To prevent an "accident," you tightly squeezed those muscles that enable you to prevent the flow of urine. These muscles surrounding the vagina are called the pubococcygeal (PC) muscles. The Kegel exercise is the tightening and relaxing of these PC muscles. To perform it you should squeeze the muscles tightly for a few seconds, then relax them. Repeat the tightening and relaxing of the muscles 10 times. This helps push any mucus at the cervix down to the vaginal opening. The Kegel exercise is excellent for keeping your vaginal muscles in shape. Not only does the exercise aid in pushing mucus down the vaginal canal, but many women feel that it also helps to increase sexual pleasure for themselves and their partners.

Other excellent times to check cervical mucus are following physical exercise or bowel movements. As with the Kegel exercise, these activities cause the mucus to travel down to the vaginal opening.

OBSERVING THE CERVIX

If you wish to learn about your cervical changes, it can be done at the same time that you check your cervical mucus.

The changes in the cervix are felt by taking the following steps (see Figure 19):

1. Wash your hands before checking the cervix to avoid the possibility of vaginal in- fection

2. Insert one or two fingers into the vaginal opening

3. Apply gentle pressure to move the finger up the vaginal canal. When the finger has reached the back of the vagina, the cervix can be felt. It is smooth, round, and feels firmer than the tissue of the vagina that surrounds it

4. As you feel the cervix, answer the following questions:
   — Is it easy or difficult to reach the cervix? In other words, is the cervix low or high in the vaginal canal?

— Does the cervix feel firm like the tip of a nose? Does it feel soft like the lips of a mouth?

— Does the opening feel closed, like a small dimple? Does it feel open, like a small hole?

5. The cervix should be checked often during the day, if possible. If this is not possible, it should be checked at least once in the morning and once in the evening

6. Squatting, or standing with one foot on a stool are good positions for cervical checking. The same position should be used each time the cervix is checked

7. It may be difficult to learn about cervical changes if you have never seen your cervix. Therefore, you can ask your clinician to show you your cervix by using a mirror. If you are not comfortable seeing

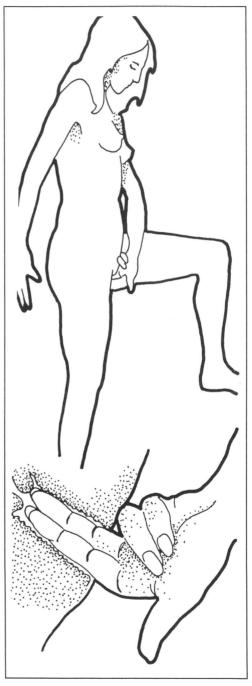

Figure 19 Checking of the Cervix

your cervix, the clinician can draw a picture of your cervix or show you a picture of a cervix.

Although the combination of cervical mucus and basal body temperature changes provides enough information to identify the fertile and infertile days accurately, some women have found observing cervical changes to be valuable in helping them determine these days.

TO REVIEW

Cervical Changes

- Relax and find the best position

- Feel the opening of the cervix

- Is the cervix difficult or easy to reach (high or low)?

- Is it soft or firm?

- Is it opening or closing as compared to the last check?

BASAL BODY TEMPERATURE OBSERVATION

The third primary fertility sign to observe is your basal body temperature (BBT). Ideally, you should use a basal body temperature thermometer. This is a special thermometer that is marked in 0.1° (1/10°) Fahrenheit or 0.05° (1/20°) Centigrade, allowing greater accuracy in measuring basal body temperature changes. Although a fever thermometer can be used, it is usually marked in 0.2° (2/10°) Fahrenheit. Since the basal body temperature thermometer provides a more accurate reading, you will probably achieve better results by using one. If you are unable to purchase a basal body temperature thermometer, a fever thermometer may do.

This is how you take your temperature:

1. Take your temperature as soon as you awaken, before you get out of bed or engage in any kind of activity

2. Take your temperature either orally (under your tongue), rectally (in your rectum), or vaginally (in your vagina) for

five minutes. Since it is important to be consistent, use the same method each time you take your temperature.

Many women find that taking their temperature orally is most convenient. However, sinus or breathing problems may require that you take your temperature vaginally or rectally.

It must be remembered that temperatures taken vaginally and rectally are about 1˚F or 0.5˚C higher than oral temperatures. Therefore, taking your temperature rectally or vaginally one day and orally another day will not provide an accurate account of the temperature pattern.

If for some reason you have to take your temperature differently one day, be sure to make a note of this on your fertility awareness chart.

3. Once the five minutes are up, read the thermometer and record your temperature on the chart. If you feel like going back to sleep after taking your temperature, put the thermometer in a safe place and read it later. Be careful not to place it near a heater, a lamp, or on a sunny ledge since the reading could easily be affected by the heat.

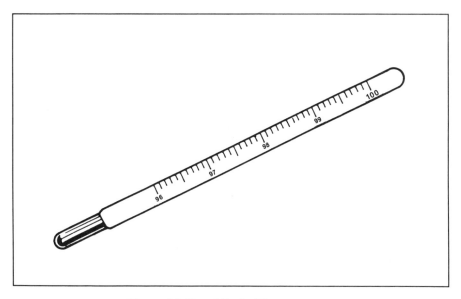

Figure 20 Basal Body Thermometer

4. Once the temperature is recorded, the thermometer should be shaken down and placed safely in its case, available for use the next day.

5. Take your temperature about the same time every day. This guarantees a more accurate temperature pattern throughout the menstrual cycle. However, if you oversleep one day or need to awaken earlier than usual another day, take your temperature when you wake up and record it. An occasional early or late temperature will probably not affect your ability to use the temperature for family planning.

6. When the temperature is recorded daily, it is important to make note of anything that may cause the temperature to be unusual. For example, taking the temperature in a different manner than usual, drinking alcoholic beverages the night before, taking a medication or a drug, awakening later or earlier than usual, or a restless night's sleep may make the temperature abnormally high or low. These events may not cause a change, but as long as they have been recorded, if they do affect your temperature you can make adjustments for them.

7. If the mercury in the thermometer is between two lines, the lower of the two temperatures is recorded. For example, if the mercury reads between 97.1˚F and 97.2˚F, the 97.1˚F reading is recorded as the temperature for the day.

8. Regardless of how the temperature is taken, you should try not to fall asleep with the thermometer in place. Rolling over may break it. The thermometer could also fall out of place, causing an inaccurate reading for the day.

USING THE BBT THERMOMETER

Place the rounded mercury end of the thermometer under your tongue. Try to put it in the same area each day since some areas of the mouth are warmer than others. Keep your lips closed over the thermometer *or*

Place the first half-inch of the thermometer in the rectum (Putting Vaseline or an oil on the tip of the thermometer makes inserting a rectal thermometer more comfortable)

or

Place the first half-inch of the thermometer into the vaginal opening (Do not use any type of lubrication—oil or jelly—since these can affect the mucus check)

TO REVIEW

Basal Body Temperature

- Use a basal body temperature thermometer

- Take your temperature just after you wake up

- Do not engage in any activity before you take your temperature—no smoking, eating, drinking or sexual activity

- Take your temperature at the same time each day

- Keep the thermometer in place for 5 minutes

These temperature-taking instructions should be followed as closely as possible. If an unexpected situation occurs—you need to go to the bathroom, care for a child, or answer a phone call—you should take your temperature as soon as you are able to.

Remember, your basal body temperature is the body temperature at rest, unaffected by activity—drinking, smoking, eating, etc. For the woman who works evenings or nights, the temperature should be taken after her usual time of sleeping.

For some women, the basal body temperature is difficult to observe because it requires awakening at about the same time every day. On the other hand, some women find that taking their temperature is not difficult, and it is a good time to relax and plan their day's activities. It has helped others to establish a routine of getting up earlier so that they have time for breakfast or an exercise routine they have wanted to enjoy.

If you are unable to take your temperature upon awakening and at the same time, you can try this: Take your temperature at the same time every night between 8 P.M. and midnight, after one hour of relaxing (putting your feet up and taking it easy!).

This way of taking the temperature works well for some women.

A LAST WORD ABOUT
OBSERVING FERTILITY SIGNS

If you feel that observing your fertility signs might be difficult for you, remember that once you feel comfortable and familiar with your fertility pattern, *you will not have to take your temperature and check your cervical mucus and cervix every day.* In fact, as soon as you enter your infertile time after ovulation, you can put the thermometer away and stop checking your temperature and other fertility signs until your next menstrual cycle begins.

YOUR NOTES:

_____

_____

_____

_____

_____

_____

_____

_____

_____

Chapter 8

Charting the Way to Awareness

The first step in learning about your fertility pattern is to observe your fertility signs. The next step is to record them on a fertility awareness chart. You will then have a visual story of each fertility cycle.

RECORDING CERVICAL MUCUS CHANGES ON THE FERTILITY AWARENESS CHART

Figure 21 shows a typical fertility awareness chart. The following five symbols are used for recording cervical mucus changes on the chart:

1. **✳** — represents menstrual bleeding.

2. **D** — represents dry days. These are the days when mucus is not present and the outside of the vagina feels dry.

3. **M** — represents sticky, pasty, and crumbly mucus that may feel slightly moist but does not feel obviously wet. The outside of the vagina feels dry.

4. **Ⓜ**— represents wet mucus. These are the days when wet-feeling mucus is present and the outside of the vagina feels wet. The mucus can be creamy or slippery and stretchy. Sometimes a wet sensation will be noticed on the outside of the vagina, but the mucus is not yet visible. In this situation the day is still considered an **M**, a wet mucus day.

5. Ⓧ— represents the one day that is the *last day* of slippery, stretchy, and very wet-feeling mucus and wet vaginal sensations. This final day is called the *peak day*. It is important to note that the peak day is not necessarily the day when

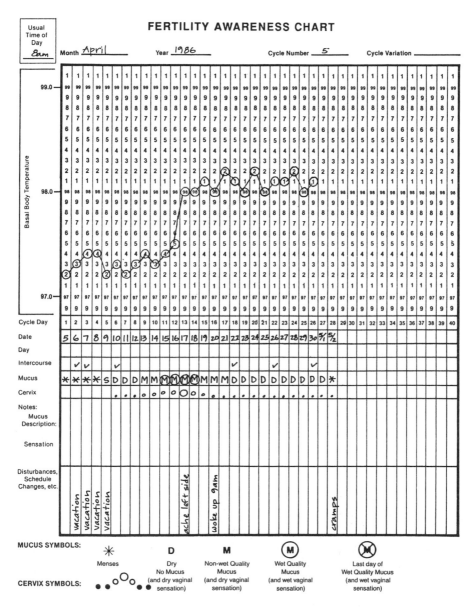

Figure 21 Recording Fertility Signs

the greatest amount of slippery, stretchy, and wet mucus is present. The peak day can only be identified the day after it has passed. It is also important to be on the lookout for this last day, especially if you are using your fertility signs as a way of preventing a pregnancy. (The Peak Day Rule is explained in Chapter 10.)

In addition to using these symbols, it can also be helpful to write down mucus descriptions in the "Notes" column on the chart. These descriptions would include the color, amount, and quality of the mucus.

Note: A blank fertility awareness chart is printed inside the back cover of this book. It can be copied on any photocopy machine and will fit on a standard 8½ x 11 inch sheet of paper. Use copies of this chart to record your personal fertility signs.

RECORDING CERVICAL CHANGES ON THE FERTILITY AWARENESS CHART

Cervical changes are recorded in the following ways:

1. A small closed circle placed in the lower left-hand corner of the box represents a low, closed cervix. [.]

2. A larger circle represents the cervix as its opening enlarges. Every day the opening feels larger, the circle becomes more open. [o]

3. As the cervix becomes higher in the vaginal canal, the circles are placed higher in the boxes. [O]

4. **S** represents a soft cervix. [O s]

5. **F** represents a firm cervix. [. F]
   S and **F** are also recorded in the boxes.

Special note: When the fertility signs are not the same throughout the day, the most fertile sign of the day is to be recorded. For example, if you have no mucus in the morning but notice a small amount of pasty mucus in the evening, the small amount of pasty mucus is recorded as the mucus of the day by using the letter **M**.

If you feel wet, creamy mucus in the morning and pasty, sticky, non-wet mucus in the evening, the wet, creamy mucus is recorded as the mucus of the day by recording **M**. If you feel the cervix in a low position in the morning and afternoon, but by evening it feels higher, the higher cervix observation is recorded, ⊡ .

RECORDING BASAL BODY TEMPERATURE (BBT) ON THE FERTILITY AWARENESS CHART

Basal body temperature (BBT) should be recorded in the temperature columns on the fertility awareness chart as follows:

1. Circle the temperature on the chart that is the same as your temperature for the day

2. Connect each circle with a straight line—this makes the changes of the temperature clear to see

3. The time you have chosen to take your temperature each day is written in the "usual time" space on the left-hand side of the chart

4. If you awaken earlier or later than usual, or experience anything else that you think might affect an accurate temperature reading, record this in the "Notes" column.

RECORDING SECONDARY FERTILITY SIGNS ON THE FERTILITY AWARENESS CHART

Secondary fertility signs are recorded as follows:

1. All physical and/or emotional changes experienced during each menstrual cycle are recorded in the "Notes" column

2. These changes should be recorded on the exact day that they are experienced

Everything and anything you feel or observe should be written down to help you learn about your own special fertility cycle.

The more information you record, the less you will need to remember, and the greater will be the rewards and discoveries you experience as your body undergoes its changes during the fertility cycle.

The key to all of the information in this book is that your body "talks" to you! It's letting you know what is occurring with your fertility cycle—a pattern of events and changes that will provide a silent but powerful personal language, the language of fertility.

Figure 21 on page 55 is an example of how to complete the fertility awareness chart.

The usual time of day the temperature is taken, and the month and year of the cycle being recorded should be noted. In this case, the usual time of temperature taking is 8:00 A.M., and the month and year of the cycle are April, 1991. The cycle number should be filled in with the number of the cycle being observed, in this case cycle number 5. Cycle variation represents the number of days in the shortest and longest cycle. In this chart, the number of days in the shortest menstrual cycle was 28 and the number of days in the longest menstrual cycle was 32. The cycle variation notation should always reflect the lengths of up to the six most recent menstrual cycles. If a woman does not know the lengths of her six most recent menstrual cycles, or if she has just discontinued taking birth control pills, had a baby, or experienced any situation that stopped ovulation, she should record her cycle lengths as she experiences them. The length of the previous menstrual cycle should be recorded as well. The fertility signs the woman chooses to observe are recorded on a daily basis along with any other descriptions of mucus, vaginal sensations, and secondary fertility signs. Any changes in lifestyle should be noted in the appropriate columns at the bottom of the chart. On our sample chart, on cycle days 3–6, a vacation is noted. Although a vacation may not change the menstrual cycle, it is noted just in case it does.

To review this chart:

The woman had knowledge of her previous four menstrual cycles, and this was the fifth cycle she was charting. The shortest cycle of her previous four cycles was 28 days; the longest cycle was 32 days. Therefore, her cycle variation up to this point is 28/32. The next chart she records will be cycle number 6. Since this cycle was 27 days long, her cycle variation on her next chart would be noted 27/32. She usually takes her temperature at 8:00 A.M. This is marked in the "usual time" space. In the "Notes" column, she recorded pain on her left side on day 13 of her menstrual cycle. On day 27 she experienced menstrual cramps, which she also noted. She recorded the fact that she awoke later than usual on cycle day 16. She also recorded the days she had intercourse by placing a "✔" in the column marked intercourse.

Please note that the more complete a chart is, the better able a woman is to apply the natural family planning rules accurately.

YOUR NOTES:

_____

_____

_____

_____

_____

_____

_____

_____

_____

Chapter 9

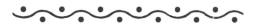

Achieving A Pregnancy & Facts About Fertility

Many have mistakenly assumed a woman can become pregnant at any time during her menstrual cycle. However, as you have learned from previous chapters, a woman has only a few fertile days when pregnancy is possible.

Therefore, if a couple want to have a baby, they must have intercourse during the fertile phase of the menstrual cycle.

INSTRUCTIONS FOR PLANNING A PREGNANCY

Ideally, you should take the time to observe your fertility signs (at least cervical mucus and basal body temperature) for a month or more before you want to achieve a pregnancy. By doing this you will become familiar with your changing mucus and temperature patterns. Knowing these patterns can help you to become familiar with your fertile days, and will enable you to determine them during future menstrual cycles. In addition, if you learn about your fertility patterns before pregnancy, you can develop the understanding necessary to use your fertility signs to avoid pregnancy after the baby is born.

Once you have observed your fertility signs for at least one menstrual cycle, *you should begin having intercourse on the first day of the wet vaginal feelings and wet mucus.* Continue having intercourse every day or every other day until the day after the temperature rises.

Having intercourse close to the time of the rise in your basal body temperature gives you the greatest possibility of pregnancy. However, since you cannot predict the exact day that your temperature will rise, *the wet cervical mucus is the best indicator of the beginning of the fertile time.* If you are observing your cervical changes, a high, soft, and open cervix is another indication of your fertile days.

Once your temperature rises, you should continue taking it for the remainder of the cycle. If your basal body temperature remains high longer than 20 days, and you don't experience your usual menstrual bleeding, it can mean that you are pregnant. If this occurs, it is important that you have a pregnancy test and be examined so that the pregnancy can be confirmed and the date the baby will be born can be determined. Another reason for this examination is the need to begin early obstetrical care for the health of the mother and baby.

TO REVIEW

- Observe your fertility signs for one cycle or more. If you want to learn about the mucus pattern, abstinence from intercourse or use of a non-lubricated condom during these cycles will enable accurate observation of the mucus changes.

- Once you've decided to become pregnant, intercourse should take place once the wet, fertile mucus begins.

- Continue taking your basal body temperature after the rise. A temperature which remains elevated beyond the usual cycle length is an excellent sign that pregnancy has been achieved.

- Having intercourse every other day maximizes the number of sperm in the semen. However, this timing of intercourse is not always necessary.

ACHIEVING CONCEPTION

If a man has no reason to suspect that he has a fertility problem, or if his semen analysis is normal, having intercourse every day during the fertile time does not seem to decrease a couple's chance for pregnancy. However, some men have a low sperm count or a problem related to the sperm movement. In this situation it is advisable for the couple to have intercourse every other day during the fertile time. This maximizes the number of sperm in the semen.

Intercourse must occur during wet mucus days to achieve pregnancy, but it doesn't mean intercourse shouldn't take place during other days in the cycle. Some couples "trying to become pregnant" change their usual sexual lifestyle in a way that isn't pleasing to them. Instead of enjoying each other sexually whenever they desire, they abstain from intercourse and from other ways of being affectionate during infertile times of the menstrual cycle.

There is no reason why intercourse can't take place at any time early in the menstrual cycle. However, since you want to be able to detect the first day of wet mucus and a wet vaginal sensation, having intercourse every other day will enable you to observe the wet mucus. Semen and wet mucus feel somewhat the same, therefore abstinence for one day after intercourse provides the time needed for semen to leave the vaginal area. This will enable a woman to accurately determine the beginning of the wet mucus production.

In addition to learning fertility signs and proper timing for intercourse, the couple desiring a pregnancy should consider a few other issues.

First, it is important to have a complete medical checkup before becoming pregnant. This examination gives you and your doctor an opportunity to discuss any medical problems that might exist. For example, if you are taking medications, it is important to know if they will be harmful if taken during pregnancy. An examination will also provide the opportunity, if necessary, for certain tests to be performed, such as for rubella (German measles), sickle cell anemia and Tay-Sachs Disease.

Another issue is selection of the child's sex through special methods of timing intercourse. Several sources have stated that pregnancy occurring as a result of intercourse a few days before the thermal shift (in other words, when wet mucus first appears) increases the possibility of the baby being a girl. Intercourse occurring near the day of the thermal shift and/or day of the most abundant wet, slippery mucus increases the possibility of a boy.

Although studies have been conducted and books have been written on this subject, planning the child's sex seems to have been successful for only a small percentage of couples. (See the Bibliography for books about selecting the sex of a baby.)

INFERTILITY

Approximately 15% of all couples have some difficulty achieving a pregnancy. Unfortunately, many of them don't know when to seek medical attention, and they are unaware of the facts about infertility tests and treatments. Other couples delay seeking medical attention because of fear. They are fearful of having a problem that cannot be corrected. Some are not aware that there are successful treatments for many causes of infertility.

On the average, it takes a couple 3–4 months to achieve a pregnancy. About 85% of couples attempting to achieve a pregnancy will succeed after one year of "trying." There are many reasons why the other 15% do not succeed. Some causes are related to problems with the man, others to problems with the woman. Sometimes, both partners will have problems. If a couple has not achieved a pregnancy after having intercourse on the fertile days for 6–9 menstrual cycles, they should seek help from a physician who treats fertility problems.

INFERTILITY AND THE MAN

The most common problems are related either to a low number of sperm in the semen or poor activity (movement) of the sperm. The causes of these problems include:

— infection

— exposure to chemicals

— medical illnesses

— prescription and non-prescription drugs

— dilated veins in the scrotum (varicocele)

Other causes of infertility are abnormalities of the testes and the passageways necessary for the normal travel of sperm and seminal fluid. These abnormalities can be due to improperly developed parts of the reproductive system, infection, or operations on or near the reproductive organs.

The first test used to check the number and quality of sperm is called *semen analysis.* If the test is not normal, additional special tests and procedures are performed to identify the cause and possible treatment of the problem. A man's semen is often tested to determine if he is allergic to his own sperm and if the sperm are able to fertilize an egg.

INFERTILITY AND THE WOMAN

Anovulation—no ovulation or infrequent ovulation—is a common cause of infertility in women, and is often successfully treated by the use of fertility drugs. Two of the more common reasons for this are:

— disturbances in the usual ways the hormones are supposed to work

— physical and emotional stress (discussed in Chapter 10)

Allergy to the man's sperm is also a cause of infertility. Another cause is cervical problems: cervical infections or surgery performed on the cervix can lead to

— inadequate production of cervical mucus

— production of cervical mucus that may not be of the quality necessary to allow sperm to live and pass through it to reach the egg

Cervical mucus can also contain substances that inactivate the sperm, in the same manner that the body produces antibodies that inactivate bacteria and viruses when it is "fighting off" an infection or illness. A common treatment for this problem is antibiotic therapy to clear up infections.

Problems of the uterus and fallopian tubes are also causes of infertility. An infection occurring in and around the internal reproductive organs (pelvic infection) can cause scarring of the fallopian tubes. This scarring may prevent the sperm from reaching the egg or the egg from entering the tube. Sometimes this can be corrected by tubal surgery.

Endometriosis (endo-me-tree-o-sis) is a cause of infertility that occurs more often in older women who have delayed having children. It is believed the endometriosis develops when the tissue which normally lines the inside of the uterus flows up through the fallopian tubes into the area of the ovaries. The presence of this tissue can cause scarring that may prevent the sperm from reaching the egg or the egg from entering the tube. Endometriosis can be treated by surgery to remove the tissue and scarring. Hormone therapy is another treatment used to reduce growth of the endometrial tissue.

OTHER CAUSES OF INFERTILITY

Approximately 5% of all couples who have an infertility evaluation will show no identifiable cause for their infertility. Some of these couples will achieve a pregnancy at some time without treatment of any kind. For others who have particularly stressful life situations, pregnancy may occur after they have dealt successfully with their stress. Some are able to do this by themselves, while others may need to seek the assistance of a professional skilled in helping people emotionally—a psychologist, counselor, or psychiatrist.

IMPROPER TIMING OF INTERCOURSE

It may take a prolonged period of time for a couple to achieve a pregnancy simply because they are unaware of the fertile phase of the menstrual cycle. Observing fertility signs can often enable a couple to achieve a pregnancy sooner because they are aware of the woman's fertile time.

FEELINGS AND INFERTILITY

Infertility is usually an extremely difficult life situation for a couple. Since many women and men have a strong desire for a child, the couple unable to have a child of their own may experience feelings of anger and frustration, as well as guilt, depression, and sadness. These feelings can be devastating to the couple and their relationship. Because of this, it can be helpful to talk with someone who can provide support and understanding. An infertility organization, therapist, counselor, or spiritual guide can provide this support and be of benefit to couples working through this very difficult time.

We have chosen not to discuss all of the many tests, causes, and treatments of fertility problems. This is not because we don't feel it is important—quite the opposite. A thorough discussion of infertility deserves its own book, of which there are many. Examples of such books are *Infertility Guide for the Childless Couple* by Barbara Eck Menning, and *Getting Pregnant and Staying Pregnant* by Diana Raab. (See the Bibliography for these books and others about infertility.)

There is also an organization of men and women committed to helping people with infertility problems. This organization, Resolve, has its headquarters in Boston, Massachusetts, and chapters in many major cities. For more information, contact Resolve, P.O. Box 474, Belmont, MA 02178.

SCIENTIFIC ADVANCES TO HELP COUPLES ACHIEVE PREGNANCY

At the present time, there are various products available to the public that can be used to closely predict the day of ovulation. Available in many drugstores, these ovulation predictor "kits" are based on the fact that the amount of a hormone made by the pituitary gland, called **luteinizing hormone** (LH), increases greatly approximately 24–36 hours before ovulation.

When a woman collects a sample of her urine on specific days during each menstrual cycle, and mixes the urine with a chemical included in the kits, the urine will change color. This color change indicates that a sudden increase in LH has happened and that ovulation will usually occur within 36 hours.

Some women choose to use an ovulation predictor test to help confirm that ovulation is taking place as well as to determine when intercourse is most likely to result in pregnancy.

At the present time, it is unknown whether the chances of achieving a pregnancy are greater using these tests as compared to timing intercourse when indicated by the presence of fertile mucus days.

If a woman, regardless of whether or not she is trying to prevent or achieve a pregnancy, is unsure that she is ovulating, the combined information from using one of these tests and keeping track of BBT and cervical mucus may give her the information she needs to confirm ovulation. However, it is advisable to seek the advice of a physician in these cases. No test is 100% accurate, and if a woman does not think she is ovulating it is important to find out why this is happening. Other tests for predicting ovulation in the future may be available, such as tests that measure changes in the saliva of the mouth or certain changes in the vagina.

There are also devices that may make BBT monitoring easier for some women. These include digital thermometers and micro-computers. Digital thermometers and microcomputers take the BBT in 1–3 minutes and are easy to read. Depending on the brand, they may or may not be as accurate as using a regular glass BBT thermometer.

In addition, microcomputers the size of a very small radio or in a wrist watch are available to help women identify fertile days. Again, there is no reason to believe these devices are any better than using fertility awareness information. And they are not par-ticularly helpful for women who ovulate irregularly. Mucus is!

YOUR NOTES:

_____

_____

_____

_____

Chapter 10

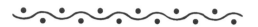

The Natural Family Planning Method

The natural family planning rules for preventing pregnancy are directions that show you how to determine the days you can have intercourse with a minimal chance of pregnancy. When accurately applied to fertility signs and followed correctly, they can provide you with an extremely safe and effective way to avoid an un-planned pregnancy.

Since there are several rules available, the ones you choose to follow will depend upon the fertility sign(s) you decide to observe and how conservative a method of NFP you want. There are rules that provide a higher effectiveness rate than others, yet require more days of abstinence than other slightly less effective rules. Though this is not an issue for some, we will discuss all the rules because others may find that the less conservative ones best meet their needs.

There are two sets of natural family planning rules:

- Those used to determine the infertile days before ovulation

- Those used to determine the infertile days after ovulation

Together the two sets of rules usually enable you to divide your menstrual cycle into three parts or phases:

1. *Phase I,* the infertile time before ovulation

2. *Phase II,* the fertile time

3. *Phase III,* the infertile time after ovulation

During the **infertile phase before ovulation,** intercourse may occur with a very small chance of pregnancy.

During the **fertile phase,** if intercourse does take place the chance of pregnancy is great.

In the **infertile phase after ovulation,** intercourse can occur with almost no chance of pregnancy.

NATURAL FAMILY PLANNING RULES USED TO DETERMINE THE INFERTILE PHASE BEFORE OVULATION: THE MOST CONSERVATIVE RULES

Rule Number 1: *Abstinence should be followed during the menstrual period.*

Surprised? If you're like many people, you learned that pregnancy could not result from having intercourse during menstruation. However, this is not always the case; although the possibility is small, (perhaps only 1–5%), it still exists. There are two basic reasons for this.

A woman can ovulate soon after her menstrual period ends. For some, this is true every menstrual cycle. These women usually have normal cycles that are less than 25 days long. For others, ovulation unexpectedly occurs earlier than usual because of a change in lifestyle, e.g., exercise or nutritional habits. This is not considered abnormal.

Your body signals you of approaching ovulation, and therefore the beginning of the fertile phase, by the appearance of cervical mucus and/or wet vaginal sensations. However, when menstrual blood is present, it is not possible to see or feel mucus. If fertile mucus is being produced during bleeding and intercourse takes place, sperm can "hang around" in the mucus for a few days, sometimes until ovulation takes place. As a result, the egg and sperm can meet and a pregnancy results.

Another reason abstinence during menstrual bleeding is advised is that some women may experience bleeding around the time they expect their menstrual period that is not menstrual bleeding! This may seem unusual, but any woman can experience bleeding as a result of a hormone imbalance or for another reason. If a woman assumes this is a normal menstrual period, has intercourse, and fertile mucus is present, she cannot detect it. Fertile mucus means ovulation is near and once again, pregnancy can result.

Some women don't enjoy intercourse during menstrual bleeding or find it objectionable for religious or other personal reasons. However, other women don't like this rule since intercourse during menstrual bleeding is pleasurable for them. If this is the case for you, you will learn later in this chapter how to determine if the bleeding you are experiencing is truly menstrual bleeding and when you can very safely have intercourse during this time with a minimal chance of pregnancy.

Rule Number 2: *Intercourse can occur during the night of any dry day. (Dry Day Rule)*

After menstrual bleeding ends, many women experience one or more dry days. Dry days are ones in which no mucus is experienced throughout the day and the vaginal sensations are dry. Because no mucus is seen, this is an indication that ovulation is probably not going to occur for several days. In addition, without the right kind of mucus, sperm cannot live and travel in the reproductive system. Therefore the possibility of pregnancy is extremely low.

The rule does state that intercourse can occur during the night of a dry day. Waiting to have intercourse until the nighttime allows you to observe for mucus and wet vaginal sensations throughout the day. It gives you ample time to make sure that no mucus is on its way down to the vaginal opening. Remember, you may not see or feel mucus in the morning, but after walking around during the day, if mucus is being produced, it will travel down to the vaginal opening and be seen later in the day.

Let's assume you take advantage of this rule and have intercourse tonight because you did not see any mucus and your vaginal sensations were dry. Tomorrow, you may experience a wet vaginal discharge. Is this discharge semen? Is it mucus? Is it a combination of both? If the wet discharge is mucus and you have intercourse again, you could become pregnant. Therefore, it is advisable to abstain from intercourse for 24 hours. If the wet discharge was semen and you were not starting to produce mucus, it will be gone within 24 hours and you will again experience a dry day. Intercourse can take place on the night of that dry day.

Having intercourse *only* on the night of a dry day, and always abstaining for 24 hours after intercourse if a wet discharge appears the next day, is a very effective rule to follow during the infertile days before ovulation.

DRY DAY RULE

Once the menstrual bleeding ends, intercourse can take place on the night of any dry day.

NATURAL FAMILY PLANNING RULE USED TO DETERMINE THE BEGINNING OF THE FERTILE PHASE

Rule Number 3: *The fertile phase begins when any type of mucus appears or wet vaginal feelings are experienced, whichever comes first. (Early Mucus Rule)*

At some point before ovulation, cervical mucus will begin to be produced. For some women, this occurs right after menstrual bleeding ends. For others, it occurs after a few dry days have passed. Regardless of when it is seen or felt, it is the signal that the egg has been maturing. There is no way of predicting early enough in advance when ovulation is going to happen. Therefore, the fertile phase begins when *any type* of mucus appears. If the vaginal feelings are wet and no mucus is seen, this is a signal that mucus is being produced and will probably be seen the next day. In either case, the fertile phase has begun. Abstinence should be followed until the fertile phase ends.

As you may have noticed, we have stated that the fertile phase begins when *any* type of mucus is seen. This means if the non-wet sticky, pasty, and crumbly mucus is seen, the fertile phase has started. This doesn't sound right, does it? Isn't fertile mucus wet? Yes! Fertile mucus is typically described as the wet-feeling mucus that often stretches and feels slippery. You might ask,"Then how can I become pregnant if the non-wet mucus is present?" The chances of pregnancy resulting from intercourse when non-wet mucus is seen is certainly small. However, it is possible. Sometimes you can see the non-wet mucus when wiping the vaginal area with toilet tissue, yet wet fertile mucus is way up in the canal of the cervix. It may take a day or so for it to flow down to the vaginal opening. Yet it's still up there, and the non-wet mucus may be a signal of this. Therefore, to be most conservative, the fertile phase begins when any type of mucus is seen. Remember, vaginal feelings can be wet, even if there is no mucus seen or the mucus is non-wet. In this situation, wet vaginal feelings are a signal that wet mucus is on the way and the fertile phase has begun.

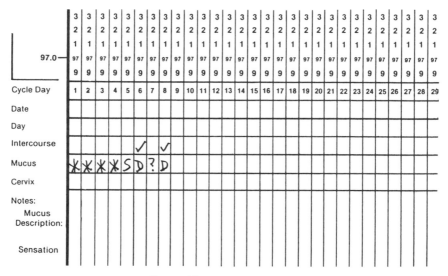

Figure 22 The Dry Day Rule

In Figure 22, a dry day was experienced on cycle day 6. Intercourse took place on that night. A wet discharge was experienced on cycle day 7. This was recorded as a question mark "?" because there was no way of determining if this discharge was mucus, semen, or a combination of both. Therefore, abstinence was followed on cycle day 7. Since cycle day 8 was a dry day, this couple decided to have intercourse that night.

It is important to note that not all women experience a wet discharge the day after intercourse. Some women have stated that if they urinate and bathe after intercourse, they don't see or feel semen in the vaginal area the next day. If this is the case and you are sure you are experiencing a completely dry day on the day following intercourse, you can have intercourse again during that night.

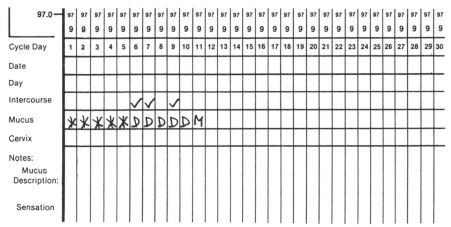

Figure 23 An example of the three rules we have just discussed

In Figure 23, Ellen experienced menstrual bleeding on cycle days 1–5. Abstinence was followed during these days. She then experienced dry days on cycle days 6–11. Ellen had intercourse on cycle day 6. This is recorded with a check mark (✔). She experienced a dry day on cycle day 7. She had intercourse again on the night of cycle day 7. Ellen could have had intercourse on cycle day 8 but chose not to. On cycle day 9 she had intercourse at night because it was a dry day. Ellen had intercourse again on the night of cycle day 10 because it was a dry day. She chose not to have intercourse on the night of cycle day 11. The fertile phase began on cycle day 12 because nonwet mucus and dry vaginal feelings were experienced on this day. Abstinence would be followed until the infertile phase after ovulation begins.

NATURAL FAMILY PLANNING RULES USED TO DETERMINE THE INFERTILE DAYS BEFORE OVULATION: LESS CONSERVATIVE RULES

The *most* conservative NFP rules to identify infertile days before ovulation are

1. Abstinence should be followed during menstrual bleeding

and

2. Intercourse can take place on the night of dry days

There are two more rules that you can use to know when you can have intercourse before the fertile phase begins. These are the Menses Rule and the Twenty-one Day Rule. Both are very effective rules (perhaps 95–99% effective), and can increase the number of days available for intercourse.

Rule Number 4: *Intercourse can occur during the first five days of the menstrual cycle. (Menses Rule)*

The Menses Rule states that the first 5 days of the menstrual cycle are safe for intercourse if the woman has applied the Thermal Shift and/or Peak Day Rules during the previous cycle. This proves that ovulation has occurred, and the bleeding she has is menstrual bleeding and not bleeding due to some other reason. The Peak Day and Thermal Shift Rules are explained later in this chapter.

MENSES RULE

The first 5 days of the menstrual cycle are safe for intercourse if ovulation took place in the previous cycle.

Only the first 5 days of the menstrual cycle are safe for intercourse. This means that if a woman's menstrual bleeding lasts for 3 days, the first 5 days are safe for intercourse. If bleeding lasts for 6 days, only the first 5 days are safe for intercourse. For those women who are comfortable having intercourse during their menstrual bleeding, this rule provides days early in the cycle when the possibility of pregnancy is extremely low.

After menstrual bleeding ends, you can use the Dry Day Rule. This rule is an excellent one for those women who wish to observe their mucus. By using this rule women can know when to have intercourse safely before the egg is released and before the fertile mucus is around to keep sperm alive. However, some women ask, "Is there another way I can know when my fertile time is going to begin, whether or not I am observing mucus?" There is a way! Women who do not want to observe mucus or who want to know in advance when their fertile phase is probably going to begin, can use the Twenty-one Day Rule. This rule got its name because it is a simple mathematical formula that gives the length of the infertile time before ovulation.

Rule Number 5: *The number of days in the infertile phase before ovulation is found by subtracting 21 from the shortest of the six most recent menstrual cycles.*

This is how to apply the rule: Find the shortest menstrual cycle that you have had in the last six cycles. You do not need to have kept a record of your fertility signs for these six cycles, you need to know only when the cycles began in order to use this rule. Subtract 21 from your shortest cycle. By doing this you will have the number of days in your infertile phase before ovulation.

For example, let's say Susan marks on her calendar when she began menstruating for the last six cycles. She finds that her cycles varied from 29–32 days in length, and the shortest cycle was 29 days. She subtracts 21 from 29, to get 8 (29-21=8). Therefore, Susan's infertile phase before ovulation is 8 days long. She can have intercourse from the first day of her menstrual cycle up to and including the eighth day of her cycle with a minimum chance of pregnancy.

TWENTY-ONE DAY RULE

The infertile phase before ovulation begins on the first day of menstruation. Its length is found by subtracting 21 from the shortest of the six most recent and consecutive normal menstrual cycles.

In another example, Ann's menstrual cycles during the months of December through May (six cycles) were 28–30 days long. If she subtracts 21 from the shortest of these cycles (28 days), she has an infertile phase of 7 days (28-21=7). So, Ann has the first 7 days of her menstrual cycle to have intercourse.

The fertile phase begins the day after this infertile phase ends. In Ann's case, since the infertile phase ended on day 7, her fertile phase began on day 8. Her fertile phase will continue until she can successfully apply the Thermal Shift and Peak Day Rules.

Why is the number 21 used to determine the length of the infertile phase before ovulation? Usually the greatest number of days that occur from ovulation to the end of the cycle is 16. The longest time that sperm may survive in fertile mucus is 5 days. Of course, 16+5=21. Subtracting 21 from the shortest menstrual cycle gives the number of days that are very safe for intercourse during the early part of the menstrual cycle.

Remember, use this rule only if:

1. You can recall accurately when your last six cycles began

   or

2. You have kept a record of the beginning of your last six cycles

   or

3. You have been charting your fertility signs for six cycles.

To apply the Twenty-one Day Rule, follow these requirements carefully:

1. Use the most recent six cycles

2. They must be normal cycles (for example, not birth control pill cycles, and they should be within the normal range of 25–37 days long)

An important factor in applying this rule is the use of the most recent six cycles to determine the infertile phase. For example, if for six cycles you never experienced a menstrual cycle shorter than 30 days, but then your seventh menstrual cycle was 28 days long, you must change your infertile phase. When your cycles were 30 days long, your infertile phase was 9 days in length (30-21=9). However, now that you have had a 28-day menstrual cycle, your infertile phase would be 7 days long. The length of a woman's menstrual cycle can normally vary a few days. If this happens to you, always make sure you use the shortest of the six most recent menstrual cycles to determine your infertile phase.

The use of the rule is about 95–99% effective in avoiding pregnancy. The small 1–5% pregnancy rate is due to the fact that the rule does not take into account an unexpected early ovulation. *The warning sign of an early ovulation is cervical mucus.* If the woman is having intercourse whenever she wants during her

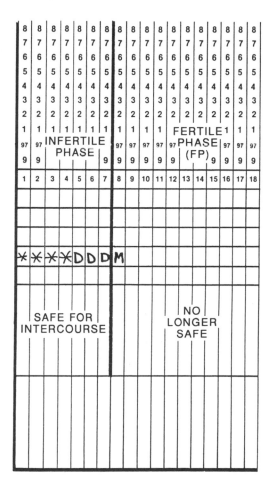

Figure 24 Infertile Phase Before Ovulation

In Figure 24, Margo's previous six menstrual cycles were 28 days in length. By subtracting 21 from 28, we see she has an infertile phase of 7 days. She can have intercourse from the first day of the menstrual cycle up to and including cycle day 7 with a minimal chance of pregnancy. Since her infertile phase ends on cycle day 7, her fertile phase begins on cycle day 8. She would then abstain until her infertile phase after ovulation begins.

infertile phase before ovulation, semen is present in the vagina. Therefore, she may not be able to see the warning mucus. If she continues to have intercourse and ovulates earlier than usual, pregnancy can occur.

For example, Joan's menstrual cycles for the past two years have been 30–32 days long. Her infertile phase before ovulation is 9 days long (30-21=9). For the first 9 days of her cycle, Joan has had intercourse whenever she desired and has not become pregnant. In one menstrual cycle Joan ovulated early. She was not aware of it because she was not watching her mucus sign, which would have been the signal for the early ovulation. She continued to have intercourse when mucus was present and became pregnant.

Is there a way of decreasing the chance of pregnancy during the infertile phase when using the Twenty-one Day Rule? There is if the Dry Day Rule is followed. When a woman can calculate the length of her infertile phase before ovulation by using the Twenty-one Day Rule, she also has the choice of using the Dry Day Rule,

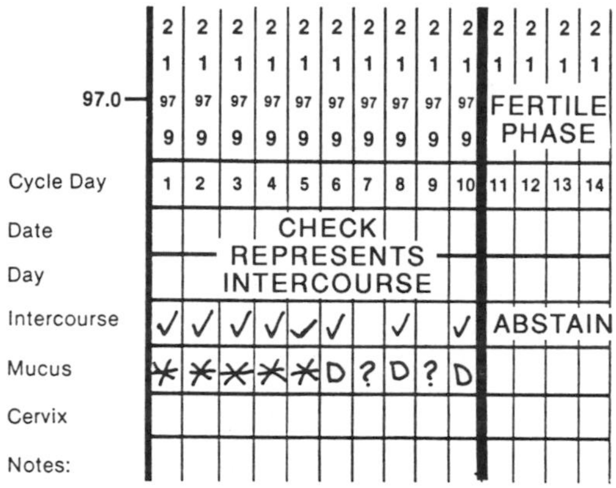

	2	2	2	2	2	2	2	2	2	2	2	2	2	2
	1	1	1	1	1	1	1	1	1	1	1	1	1	1
97.0	97	97	97	97	97	97	97	97	97	97	FERTILE			
	9	9	9	9	9	9	9	9	9	9	PHASE			
Cycle Day	1	2	3	4	5	6	7	8	9	10	11	12	13	14
Date			CHECK											
Day		REPRESENTS INTERCOURSE												
Intercourse	√	√	√	√	√	√		√		√	ABSTAIN			
Mucus	✳	✳	✳	✳	✳	D	?	D	?	D				
Cervix														
Notes:														

Figure 25 The Twenty-one Day Rule, Menses Rule, and Dry Day Rule

In Figure 25, Naomi's last six cycles were 31 days long. Therefore, her infertile phase before ovulation is 10 days long. Because she would like to minimize the chance of pregnancy as much as possible while having intercourse before ovulation, she used the Menses Rule and Dry Day Rule during her infertile phase. By applying the Menses Rule, the first 5 days were safe for intercourse. Since she was still bleeding on cycle day 4, she could not observe possible mucus. On cycle day 6 she experienced a dry day. By using the Dry Day Rule, she had intercourse on the evening of that day. She abstained throughout cycle day 7 to allow semen to leave the vaginal area. On cycle day 8 she continued to abstain until she was sure the entire day was dry again. Because it was, she had intercourse on that evening. She abstained on cycle day 9 again and because cycle day 10 was dry the entire day, it was still safe for intercourse. Since her infertile phase ended on day 10, her fertile phase began on day 11. On cycle day 11 she began her period of abstinence.

which will enable her to see her body signaling her that her ovulation is going to happen earlier than usual. The early warning mucus is that body signal. A woman can also choose to abstain during menstrual bleeding or use the Menses Rule. It all depends upon how conservative a method of family planning she wants.

Caution: If any mucus is detected within the infertile phase before ovulation, the woman must consider herself potentially fertile since the mucus may indicate an early ovulation.

NATURAL FAMILY PLANNING RULES USED TO DETERMINE THE INFERTILE PHASE AFTER OVULATION

Rule Number 6: The infertile phase after ovulation begins on the evening of the fourth day after the peak day. (Peak Day Rule)

The Peak Day Rule is the rule applied to the cervical mucus. It is called the Peak Day Rule because the peak day must be identified in order to use this rule.

As you recall, usually within a few days after the menstrual flow ends, cervical mucus will be observed. As ovulation nears, this mucus will become very wet, slippery, and stretchy, causing a wet feeling in the vaginal area. At some point after ovulation the mucus will lose its slippery, stretchy, and wet quality, and the wet vaginal sensations will no longer be present. *The last day of the wet vaginal feelings and slippery, stretchy, wet mucus is the peak day.* To identify the peak day you will be looking for the first day the wet vaginal feeling is no longer present and the mucus feels significantly drier. (Some women notice that they stop having mucus after the peak day and for the remainder of the menstrual cycle.) As you can see, the peak day can be identified only *after* it has taken place. For example, you may experience slippery, stretchy, and wet mucus and wet vaginal feelings Monday through Friday; then on Saturday you observe a mucus that is no longer slippery, stretchy, and wet, or considerably less wet than it has been, and the wet vaginal feelings are gone. This means that Friday, the last day of your wet feelings followed by a significantly drier feeling mucus that is no longer stretchy, is your peak day.

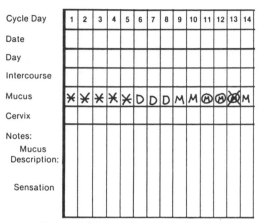

Cycle Day	1	2	3	4	5	6	7	8	9	10	11	12	13	14
Date														
Day														
Intercourse														
Mucus	*	*	*	*	*	D	D	D	M	M	Ⓜ	Ⓜ	Ⓜ (X)	M
Cervix														
Notes: Mucus Description:														
Sensation														

Figure 26 Identifying the Peak Day

In Figure 26, Joanne has recorded 5 days of menstrual bleeding. Once the bleeding ended, she began observing for mucus. On cycle days 6, 7, and 8, because no mucus was observed and a dry vaginal feeling was experienced, these days were recorded as dry days. On cycle days 9 and 10 she experienced a pasty, sticky mucus with a dry vaginal feeling. Joanne began producing wet, slippery, and stretchy mucus on cycle day 11. These wet days continued until cycle day 13. On cycle day 14 she noticed that her wet feelings were no longer present. She felt a dry feeling and had sticky, pasty mucus. At this point she was able to go back to the last day of wet, slippery, and stretchy mucus and wet feelings and mark it as her peak day. Placing an X through the circled M represented the peak day for that cycle.

PEAK DAY RULE

The infertile phase after ovulation begins on the evening of the fourth consecutive day of sticky, pasty, and crumbly mucus and/or dry days after the peak day.

As you have probably noticed, we continuously reinforce vaginal feelings. Remember that the vaginal feelings experienced are dependent upon the quality of the mucus present. Wet mucus causes a wet vaginal feeling, and a total absence of mucus or sticky, pasty, and crumbly mucus causes a dry vaginal feeling.

If you feel a wet feeling but don't see wet mucus, your peak day has not yet occurred. You have experienced the last day of

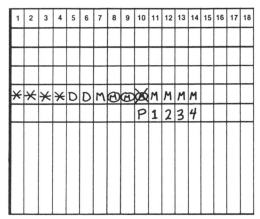

Figure 27 The Peak Day Rule

In Figure 27, on cycle day 11 Marlene no longer experienced wet vaginal feelings, and her mucus felt less wet than it had on cycle days 8, 9, and 10. Because of this she could mark cycle day 10, the last wet day, as her peak day. Marlene could then apply the peak day rule because she experienced 4 days of sticky, pasty mucus and dry vaginal feelings in a row after her peak day. Her infertile phase after ovulation began on the evening of cycle day 14.

---

wetness—the peak day—only when both the mucus and vaginal feelings are no longer wet.

Once the peak day is determined, the rule can be applied.

Remember, ovulation can occur any time up to 3 days before the peak day to one day after the peak day. Waiting until the evening of the fourth day to resume intercourse provides sufficient time for the release and life span of the egg. When the infertile phase begins, you no longer need to observe your mucus.

Caution: *Occasionally a woman experiences the reappearance of slippery, stretchy, and wet mucus after she has identified what she believed to be her peak day. She will know it was not her peak day because instead of having 4 sticky, pasty, and crumbly mucus and/or dry days in a row, wet mucus reappears. If this happens, abstinence should be continued until the true peak day is identified and the wetness is absent for 4 days in a row.*

There are two common reasons for the reappearance of wet mucus. First, a woman may identify her peak day improperly.

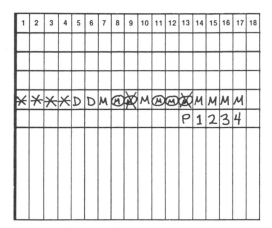

Figure 28 Identifying the True Peak Day

In Figure 28, Ruth thought her peak day occurred on cycle day 9 since on cycle day 10 she experienced a sticky, pasty mucus with dry vaginal feelings. However, while waiting for the 4 days to pass, she noticed a reappearance of wet mucus. She realized that either she had made an error in identifying her peak day or perhaps she was ovulating later than usual. She continued to abstain and waited until her wet mucus production stopped. She then identified a peak day on cycle day 13. This time she was correct, because she then experienced sticky, pasty mucus days with dry vaginal feelings for 4 days in a row. Therefore, according to the Peak Day Rule, her infertile phase began the evening of cycle day 17.

However, the greater her experience with mucus observations, the less likely this is. Second, ovulation can be delayed. A delay in ovulation can cause wet mucus to come and go until the egg is finally released. These situations need not be a problem if two key points are remembered:

1. Always wait until the evening of the fourth sticky, pasty, and crumbly mucus and/or dry day after the peak day to resume intercourse. Vaginal feelings must be dry during these four days.

2. Always wait to resume intercourse until the Thermal Shift Rule is applied (Rule Number 7).

The temperature pattern can help you greatly if these situations occur, since the peak day usually occurs around the same time as the thermal shift. This means that the beginning of the infertile phase is usually the same when the Thermal Shift and Peak Day Rules are applied. *If the two rules do not coincide, the more conservative rule must be followed before resuming intercourse.*

For example, if you have applied the Thermal Shift Rule and it gives you an infertile phase beginning Wednesday evening, yet application of the Peak Day Rule gives you an infertile phase beginning on Tuesday evening, these two rules do not coincide. To be sure you are no longer fertile, use the more conservative rule. In this example, intercourse should not begin on Tuesday evening but on Wednesday evening.

Rule Number 7: The infertile phase after ovulation begins on the night of the third consecutive temperature recorded above the coverline. (Thermal Shift Rule)

The Thermal Shift Rule is the rule that is applied to the basal body temperature. It is called the Thermal Shift Rule because you will be on the lookout for a shift in temperature. A shift is a change (a rise) from the low temperatures occurring before ovulation to the higher temperatures occurring shortly before, during or shortly after ovulation. The basal body temperatures will shift upward usually 0.3˚–1˚F or 0.15˚–0.6˚C higher than the low temperatures recorded up to that point. This usually happens the same day or one to two days after the egg is released.

To apply the Thermal Shift Rule, follow these steps:

1. After you have recorded temperatures from cycle days 1–10, look at these temperatures and locate the highest one you have recorded.

2. Draw a line across your chart that is just 0.1˚F or .05˚C above the highest temperature you recorded during the first ten days of the menstrual cycle. This line is called the **coverline**.

3. Continue to take your basal body temperature. At some point, the temperatures will rise above the coverline.

4. Once this happens, your infertile phase after ovulation will begin on the night of the third consecutive temperature recorded above the coverline.

THERMAL SHIFT RULE

The infertile phase after ovulation begins on the evening of the third consecutive day of temperatures recorded above the coverline.

The egg will only live for 24 hours unless it is fertilized. Waiting to resume intercourse until the evening of the third day allows sufficient time for the release and life span of one, and perhaps two, eggs. If an egg is no longer present, there can be no pregnancy!

Caution: If any one of the three temperatures falls on or below the coverline, it can be a sign that ovulation has not yet taken place. Therefore, wait until the temperatures rise back above the coverline and then apply the 3-day count again.

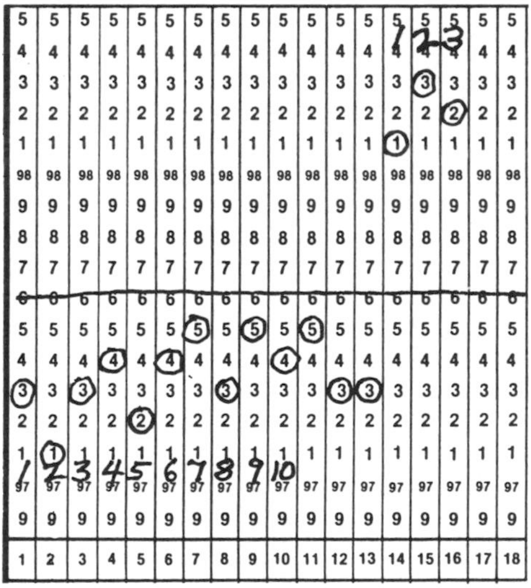

Figure 29 The Thermal Shift Rule

In Figure 29, the temperature shifted to 98.1°F on cycle day 14. To draw the coverline, we first look at the ten temperatures. Next, we find the highest of the ten temperatures. In this case it is 97.5°F. Finally, by adding ¹⁄₁₀ of a degree to 97.5°F, we can draw the coverline at 97.6°F. Waiting for three temperatures in a row to be recorded above the coverline gives us an infertile phase beginning on the evening of cycle day 16.

FALSE HIGH RISES

Occasionally, around the time of ovulation, you may observe a rise in temperature and assume it is your thermal shift. However, instead of remaining above the coverline for three consecutive days, the temperature may fall back on or below it. Therefore, the temperature rise was for a reason other than ovulation. This is called a false high rise. A false high rise can be caused by over-sleeping one day or by experiencing one of the situations discussed in Chapter 7 that can cause an unusual temperature rise. False high rises, as we have stated, cannot be used when applying the Thermal Shift Rule. Always use only those high temperatures which reflect accurate normal basal body temperatures.

A false high temperature can also occur early in the menstrual cycle. For example, some women experience high temperatures during menstruation. By the time bleeding ends, the temperatures have returned to low levels again. However, this will not prevent you from correctly applying the Thermal Shift Rule. For example, if one of the 10 temperatures before the rise is high instead of low, it would not be used to determine the coverline. However, it would still be included when counting the first ten days.

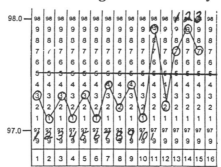

Figure 30 Identifying the True Thermal Shift

In Figure 30, the temperature shifted to 97.9°F on cycle day 11. The coverline was drawn at 97.5°F which is 1/10 of a degree above the highest of the first ten low temperatures. As you can see, the temperature dropped back down below the coverline. Therefore, we have to wait until the true shift in temperature takes place to determine the beginning of the infertile phase. The temperature rises again on cycle day 13. We know this is the true thermal shift because the temperature stays above the line for 3 days in a row. Therefore, in this example the infertile phase begins on the evening of cycle day 15

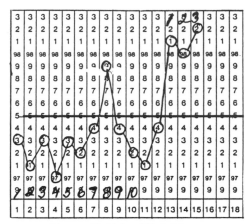

Figure 31 False High Rise

In Figure 31, the temperature rises on cycle day 8. Because the rise had taken place in the early part of Jane's menstrual cycle, before she usually experiences her thermal shift, she knew this rise was probably not her real thermal shift. She also overslept that morning and took her temperature a couple of hours later than usual. (Although she could be experiencing an unexpected early ovulation, she was not producing any cervical mucus. If she were ovulating early, she would be able to observe the early warning sign of mucus.) She continued to take her temperature and found that it shifted on cycle day 13. She drew her coverline 1/10 of a degree above the highest of the first ten temperatures of her cycle before the thermal shift. Since the temperature on cycle day 8 was unusually high, it was not counted as one of the ten temperatures recorded, but would not be used to draw the coverline.

Occasionally, after menstruation ends there may be more than two high temperatures experienced during the remaining days up to and including day 10. This can reflect improper temperature taking or perhaps an unusual menstrual cycle. If this should happen, we suggest continuing abstinence until you can discuss this irregular basal body temperature with someone very experienced in the use of fertility signs.

One more situation to discuss regarding the Thermal Shift Rule is that of early ovulation. A woman who ovulates early in her cycle will experience a thermal shift before ten temperatures have been recorded. When this occurs the woman should draw a coverline 0.1°F above the highest temperatures recorded up to that point. Once this is done, the Thermal Shift Rule can be applied.

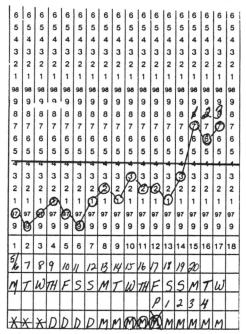

Figure 32 Use the Most Conservative Rule

In Figure 32, Sheri applied both the Peak Day Rule and Thermal Shift Rule. The Peak Day Rule gave her an infertile phase beginning on the evening of cycle day 16. However, the Thermal Shift Rule gave an infertile phase beginning on the evening of cycle day 17. To be safe, Sheri used the more conservative rule—in this case the Thermal Shift Rule—and her infertile phase began the evening of cycle day 17.

For example, if you experience a thermal shift on cycle day 9, draw a coverline 0.1°F or 0.05°C above the highest normal low temperature recorded from cycle day 1–8. Once the coverline is drawn, continue to take your temperature. Once three consecutive temperatures have been recorded above the coverline, the infertile phase after ovulation has begun.

TO REVIEW

- Find the highest normal low temperature recorded during the first 10 days of the menstrual cycle

- Draw the coverline 0.1° F or 0.05° C above the highest of the ten temperatures

- Wait for three days in a row of high temperatures above the coverline

- The evening of the third day of high temperatures is the beginning of the infertile phase after ovulation, and intercourse can be resumed until the next menstrual flow begins

- You can put your thermometer away after the beginning of the infertile phase

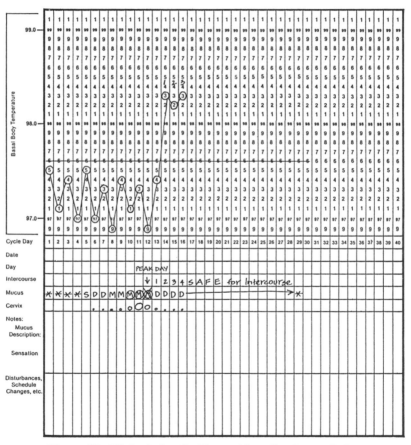

Figure 33 All the Infertile Phase After Ovulation Rules

In Figure 33, Kim observed her mucus, cervix, and basal body temperature, and by applying all the rules saw that her infertile phase began on the evening of cycle day 16. Since her menstrual cycle was 30 days long, she could safely have intercourse from the evening of the 16th day up to and including cycle day 30. During these days she no longer needed to observe her fertility signs.

Charting your basal body temperature is an accurate way of determining that you have ovulated and are no longer able to become pregnant. Remember that the temperature rises around the time of ovulation. Therefore, it makes sense to use the temperature shift in combination with the changes in cervical mucus in order to be as accurate as possible in determining the beginning of the infertile time after ovulation. Another advantage in using the basal body temperature is that it can help you make sure you have identified the peak day properly.

SUMMARY OF THE THREE PHASES
OF THE MENSTRUAL CYCLE

Phase I, the Infertile Phase Before Ovulation, includes:

1. The menstrual flow

2. Days which are dry (mucus is not present and there is a dry vaginal sensation)

3. Days in which the cervix is low, firm and closed

4. Low basal body temperatures, with the possible exception of a few higher temperatures which may occur during the menstrual flow

Phase II, the Fertile Phase, includes:

1. All mucus days until the Peak Day Rule is applied

2. Days in which the cervix is higher in the vaginal canal, and soft and open

3. The rising of the basal body temperature from low levels to high levels until the Thermal Shift Rule is applied

Phase III, the Infertile Phase After Ovulation, includes:

1. Days when mucus is pasty, sticky, and crumbly and/or days which are completely dry, and it may include a few wet days at the end of the menstrual cycle

2. Days in which the cervix is low, firm, and closed

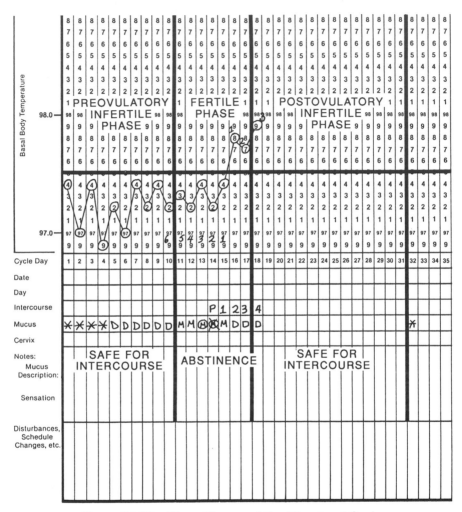

Figure 34 The Three Phases of the Menstrual Cycle

In Figure 34, Angela's last six menstrual cycles were 31 days in length. Therefore, by using the Twenty-one Day Rule, her infertile phase before ovulation is 10 days long. Depending upon the effectiveness rate she chooses, she can have intercourse whenever she desires during the infertile phase or use the Menses Rule, Dry Day Rule, or both during this infertile phase. Her fertile phase began on cycle day 11. Abstinence was observed until the infertile phase after ovulation rules could be applied. She chose to observe her mucus and basal body temperatures, but not her cervix. By application of the Thermal Shift Rule and Peak Day Rule, she could resume intercourse on the night of cycle day 18. She could then have intercourse when she wanted up to and including cycle day 31.

3. Days in which the temperature remains at a high level for about 12–16 days

SHORT CYCLE CALCULATIONS

If a woman's menstrual cycles are usually less than 25 days long, she can use the Twenty-one Day Rule to determine the length of her infertile phase before ovulation. However, to be more conservative, it is advisable that abstinence begin on the first day of menstruation.

Short cycles mean that ovulation takes place early in the cycle, a few days after the menstrual flow ends. Because of this, cervical

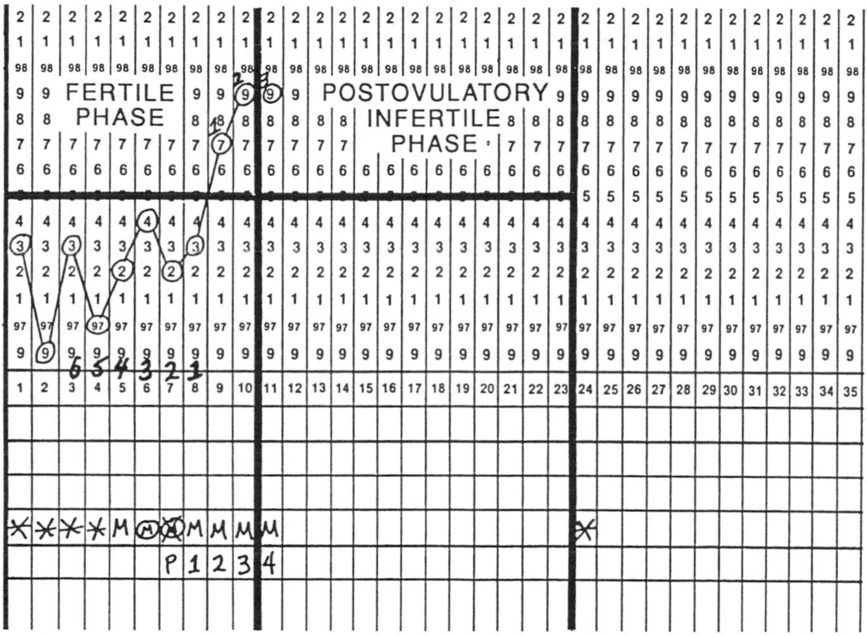

Figure 35 The Short Cycle

In Figure 35, Jade's previous 6 menstrual cycles were 23–26 days in length. Since she normally experiences short menstrual cycles, she does not have an infertile phase before ovulation. Therefore, her fertile phase begins on the first day of her menstrual cycle and ends when she can successfully apply the infertile phase after ovulation rules. In this example she had to abstain from cycle day 1 through cycle day 11. She could resume intercourse the night of cycle day 11 up to and including the end of her menstrual cycle, day 23.

mucus can be present during the menstrual flow. The bleeding makes observation of the mucus difficult if not impossible. If intercourse occurs and mucus is present, the sperm may be able to survive long enough to fertilize the egg at ovulation. The result is that for a woman with short cycles pregnancy may occur from intercourse taking place during the first few days of her menstrual cycle.

Therefore, a woman with short cycles has two instead of three phases to her menstrual cycle—a fertile phase and an infertile phase after ovulation. *The first day of menstrual bleeding is the first day of the fertile phase.* The fertile phase ends and the infertile phase after ovulation begins when the Thermal Shift Rule and Peak Day Rule have been applied.

THE BASIC INFERTILE PATTERN

There are a few women who always see mucus as soon as the menstrual flow ends, instead of experiencing dry days. These women experience the same type of mucus every day during the infertile phase before ovulation. This situation of daily non-changing mucus that does not feel wet is called a basic infertile mucus pattern. Since there are no dry days during the infertile phase before ovulation, the Dry Day Rule is applied to the non-changing mucus. In other words, the non-changing mucus days are used as though they were dry, no-mucus days. *Therefore, intercourse may occur the night of non-changing mucus days.*

These women must be careful to be on the lookout for any change in their basic infertile patterns. *If the mucus or vaginal feelings change in any way, it may mean that ovulation is approaching.* If the mucus does change, the fertile phase has started and abstinence must begin.

Caution: *A woman may need to observe her mucus for two or more menstrual cycles to develop the experience necessary to use this rule.*

A Special Note about Cervical Mucus

It is important to remember that certain factors can affect the cervical mucus, preventing the accurate observations needed to successfully apply the mucus rules. These factors are:

1. *Douching,* which removes most cervical mucus from the vaginal canal. (It does not remove all of it, which is why douching is not a successful method of birth control. However, it can remove enough of the mucus to make cervical mucus observations inaccurate).

2. *Semen* that is left in the vaginal canal after intercourse. It mixes with cervical mucus making the observation of the mucus very difficult if not impossible.

3. *Sexual arousal,* which causes moisture to form in the vaginal canal, making it difficult to determine when mucus is present. You should wait until the wet feeling from sexual arousal is gone before checking for cervical mucus.

4. *Spermicidal agents* (creams, jellies and foams), which remain in the vagina for a day or more after their use. You should not use them if you want to observe your mucus as accurately as possible.

5. *A vaginal infection,* which can prevent accurate observation of cervical mucus. The way to handle this situation is discussed further in Chapter 11.

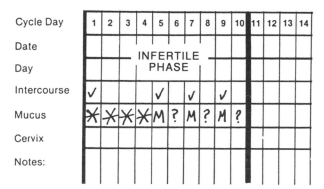

Figure 36 The Basic Infertile Pattern

In Figure 36, Cheryl had observed the same type of mucus every day for 10 days. Because she felt she had gained the experience to be confident with her mucus observations, she used the days of non-changing mucus (or her basic infertile pattern) as though they were dry days. Her fertile phase began on cycle day 11 because her mucus changed. It became slightly wet, indicating the approach of ovulation.

If you wish to use the natural family planning rules well, it is important to do the following:

- Observe your fertility signs accurately

- Chart your fertility signs and changes accurately

- Follow the rules as they have been explained

ONE MORE SITUATION TO THINK ABOUT

What should a woman do if she does not have an accurate history of her most recent six menstrual cycles or has just stopped using birth control pills? In both of these situations she does not have the proper information to use the Twenty-one Day Rule. To be most conservative and safe, the woman should consider herself fertile from the first day of menstrual bleeding until her infertile phase after ovulation begins. Once she has six cycles recorded, the Twenty-one Day rule can be used to determine the safe days early in the menstrual cycle.

However, some women find that waiting for six cycles to pass is unsatisfactory. They would like to have intercourse safely before ovulation even though they are not able to use the Twenty-one Day Rule. These women choose to use the Dry Day and Menses Rules. In other words, they can have intercourse during the first five days of the cycle, and once the bleeding ends, they begin observing their cervical mucus. If mucus is not present throughout the entire day, and dry vaginal feelings are experienced, they can have intercourse on the night of the dry day. They then continue to use the Dry Day Rule until mucus production begins. Once mucus is observed and/or the vaginal feelings are no longer dry, the fertile phase has begun. Abstinence should be followed until the start of the infertile phase after ovulation.

SYMPTO-THERMAL METHOD CHOICES

As we explained in Chapter 2, the sympto-thermal method of natural family planning combines observation of mucus, basal body temperature, and other fertility signs. The basic choices for couples using this method are:

Before Ovulation

1. A couple can abstain during menstrual bleeding

   or

   have intercourse during the first 5 days of the menstrual cycle if ovulation occurred the previous cycle. A couple can also have intercourse on the night of a dry day. These rules can be used with or without the Twenty-one Day Rule.

2. The fertile phase begins when mucus and/or wet vaginal sensations are experienced, when the Twenty-one Day Rule is applied, or whichever comes first.

After Ovulation

3. The Peak Day and Thermal Shift Rules should be followed.

USING THE CERVICAL MUCUS METHOD TO PREVENT PREGNANCY

Some women cannot or do not want to observe their basal body temperature and instead choose to follow cervical mucus changes to prevent pregnancy. Though this book is primarily devoted to discussing the sympto-thermal method, we'd like to introduce this family planning option because use of cervical mucus to prevent pregnancy is an effective method of NFP. If you would like to use the cervical mucus method, we advise reading *The Billings Method Book* by Dr. Evelyn Billings, and attending a cervical mucus method program in your area.

CERVICAL MUCUS METHOD RULES

The most conservative rules to use with mucus observations are as follows:

Rule Number 1: Intercourse should be avoided during menstrual bleeding. As previously explained in this chapter, this rule is based on the possibility that a woman may ovulate a few days after menstrual bleeding ends. When this happens, fertile cervical mucus is often being produced during menstruation. Yet a woman will probably not be able to see or feel this mucus due to the presence of blood. Therefore, she is unable to use her mucus as a signal that menstruation is a fertile time. If intercourse takes place during menstruation and fertile mucus is present, sperm may be able to live until ovulation occurs and a pregnancy can result. The possibility of ovulation occurring shortly after menstruation ends is not a common one, but it can happen. This is why the most conservative approach for the use of the cervical mucus method is to abstain during menstruation.

It is also important to note that a woman may assume she is menstruating but instead be experiencing bleeding for various reasons such as ovulation, a hormone imbalance, or a problem of the reproductive organs. If ovulation is occurring or is about to occur and a couple has intercourse, pregnancy can result. (If a woman experiences bleeding that she feels may not be menstrual bleeding, it is important to discuss this with her physician).

Option to Rule Number 1: Intercourse can take place during the first five days of the menstrual cycle if a woman has successfully applied the Peak Day Rule the previous cycle and the cycle appeared normal for her.

Rule Number 2: Intercourse can occur the night of any dry day during the infertile phase before ovulation. This is the same Dry Day Rule explained in our discussion of the sympto-thermal method rules.

Option to Rule Number 2: If the day after intercourse is dry the entire day, abstinence does not need to be followed and intercourse can once again occur on that evening.

Rule Number 3—The Early Mucus Rule: The fertile phase always begins on the first day any type of mucus is observed and/or wet vaginal sensations are experienced. This means that even if the sticky, pasty, and crumbly mucus is present, it is still an indication that a woman has probably entered her fertile time. Remember that although this mucus is typically the infertile type, when it is seen before ovulation it could be a signal that wet, slippery, and stretchy, fertile mucus is starting to be produced in the cervix but hasn't yet traveled down to the vaginal opening. Consequently, intercourse at this time could result in pregnancy.

What is the possibility of pregnancy when intercourse takes place on the days that sticky, pasty, and crumbly mucus is observed? The answer to this question is not known at the present time. Some sources state that the chances are small. However, an actual pregnancy rate based on couples having intercourse when this kind of mucus is present before ovulation has not been determined. Therefore, if you want to follow the most conservative approach, abstinence should be followed every day beginning with the first day that any type of mucus appears, and continuing until the fertile phase has ended. A less conservative approach is to have intercourse on the evening of every other day that the sticky, pasty mucus is present. When the mucus changes to a wetter quality, the fertile phase has begun.

Rule Number 4—The Peak Day Rule: The same Peak Day Rule as explained previously is used to determine the beginning of the infertile phase after ovulation.

TO REVIEW: CERVICAL MUCUS METHOD
—CONSERVATIVE APPROACH

- Abstain during menstrual bleeding.

- When menstruation ends, mucus observations should begin. If dry days are experienced, the Dry Day Rule can be followed.

- The fertile phase begins on the first day any type of mucus and/or wet vaginal sensations are experienced, whichever comes first.

- The infertile phase after ovulation begins on the evening of the fourth day after the peak day has been identified.

Now it is time for you to practice the NFP rules by using the menstrual cycle history of fertility signs that have been recorded by Alicia (Figure 37).

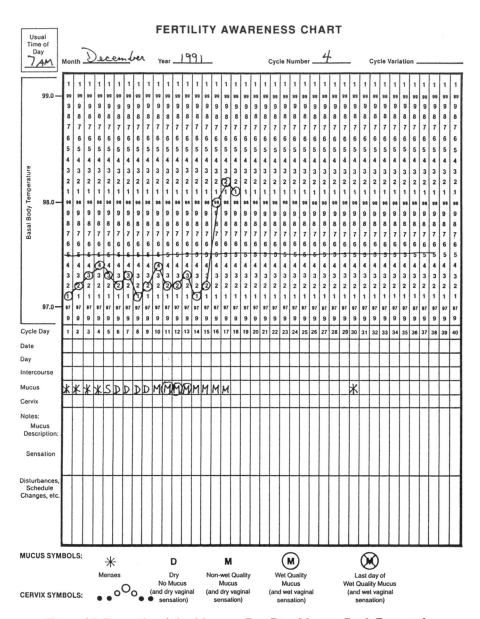

Figure 37 Example of the Menses, Dry Day, Mucus, Peak Day, and
Thermal Shift Rules

In Figure 37, Alicia has been recording her mucus and temperature for three cycles. These cycles have ranged from 28–32 days in length. She usually takes her temperature at 7A.M. Last cycle, Alicia knew she ovulated because she had a rise in her temperature and could apply the Temperature Rule. She also experienced a peak day and applied the Peak Day Rule.

1. Could Alicia have intercourse during menstrual bleeding? Yes. Since Alicia applied the Peak Day and Temperature Rules the previous menstrual cycle, she knows the bleeding she experienced this cycle is a true menstrual period. Therefore, she could have intercourse during cycle days 1–5 (Menses Rule).

2. If Alicia had intercourse on cycle day 5 (which is also a dry day) could she have intercourse on cycle day 6? Yes. Alicia did not experience any mucus and had dry vaginal sensations on cycle day 6. Therefore, intercourse could take place on the night of that day. Since Alicia experienced dry days on cycle days 7 and 8, she could again have intercourse on the night of cycle day 7 as well as on the night of cycle day 8. Remember, if Alicia had experienced a vaginal discharge on a day after intercourse, she would have to abstain for 24 hours to be able to determine if the discharge was semen, mucus, or both. If after the 24 hours of abstinence, she experienced a dry day again, intercourse could occur on that night.

3. When does the fertile phase begin? It begins on cycle day 9, since this is when Alicia experienced mucus. Though it wasn't wet mucus, wet mucus could be up in the cervix and could take a day to travel down to the vaginal opening.

4. When does the fertile phase end? To determine this, you first need to identify the peak day. This was on cycle day 12. Remember, the peak day is the last day of wet mucus and wet vaginal feelings. To apply the Peak Day Rule, Alicia must continue to abstain until four days of nonwet mucus and/or dry days are experienced after the peak day. The fertile phase ends on the night of the fourth day after the peak day, which is on cycle day 17. Intercourse can be resumed on the night of the fourth day and continue until the end of the cycle.

Alicia should also apply the temperature rule to know when the fertile phase has ended. To do this, she first needs to draw the coverline 0.1°F or 0.05°C above the highest temperature recorded during the first ten days of the cycle. Once this is done, the fertile phase ends, and the infertile phase begins on the night of the third high temperature recorded above the coverline. The night of the third high temperature is recorded on cycle day 18.

To be safe, Alicia should follow the most conservative rule. The Peak Day Rule shows that the infertile phase begins on the night of cycle day 17, but the Thermal Shift Rule shows that the infertile phase begins on the night of cycle day 18. Therefore, to be most conservative, the infertile phase begins on the night of cycle day 18. Intercourse can be resumed on this night and can continue any day, any time, until the menses begins again. Alicia no longer has to observe her fertility signs until the next cycle begins. When Alicia has recorded six cycles she can choose to use the Twenty-one Day Rule with or without checking her mucus.

SPECIAL NOTE

Use of natural family planning has no known physical side effects for the woman. However, there are a few studies that suggest, but do not prove, that couples who have had an unplanned pregnancy using periodic abstinence had a higher incidence of spontaneous abortion, as well as children born with certain mental and physical defects.

It is thought that one cause of the higher incidence of these problems may be due to the fertilization of an overripe egg. This can occur if intercourse has not taken place before ovulation but only 1–2 days after the temperature rise. This can result in fertilization of an overripe egg.

Another possible cause of these problems is due to fertilization of an egg by an overaged sperm. If during prolonged periods of abstinence from intercourse ejaculation has not taken place, overaged sperm can be present when intercourse is resumed.

We have added this information, not to alarm you, but to enable you to put this debatable issue into perspective. If an increase in spontaneous abortion and birth defects is related to the use of NFP, carefully following the infertile phase after ovulation rules would minimize this possibility. These rules allow for the release and life span of two eggs. Therefore, the chances of pregnancy when intercourse is resumed are minimal.

WHEN CAN YOU BEGIN USING THESE RULES TO AVOID PREGNANCY?

During the first cycle of observing and charting you may be able to use these rules to determine the infertile phase after ovulation. However, this can be done *only* if you are certain about what you are experiencing. If you are not, you must wait at least another menstrual cycle, until you are more comfortable with your own fertility pattern, before you apply these rules. You must be confident that you are following the instructions for checking and charting properly, and applying the rules correctly, before assuming you are no longer fertile and resuming intercourse.

YOUR NOTES:

_____

_____

_____

_____

_____

_____

_____

_____

_____

Chapter 11

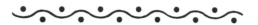

Special Circumstances: The Early Years, the Later Years, Breastfeeding, Illnesses, etc.

It is not uncommon for us to make plans which have to be changed at the last minute. Yet, the change need not ruin our day if we make room for it to happen.

This is true of the fertility cycle. Natural family planning can be used successfully with the normal ovulatory cycle, and if something happens to cause a change in the cycle or the patterns of the fertility signs, they can still be followed to avoid pregnancy.

Any situations which cause a change in your menstrual cycle or patterns of fertility signs are called special circumstances.

If special circumstances occur, you can usually continue to use fertility signs successfully to avoid pregnancy. Pregnancy can be avoided by knowing what to look for and by using the special circumstances rules explained in this chapter.

Special circumstances include

- fever

- breastfeeding

- stress

- ovarian cyst

- previous birth control pill use

- exercise

- diet

- travel

- illness

- premenopause

The most frequent special circumstances are common illnesses. The most common of these are the cold and flu. These are types of infections that can cause the body temperature to rise unusually high, which is known as a fever. When you have a fever, your basal body temperature will remain high until you begin to recover from the illness.

Having a fever need not be a difficult or confusing situation if you are using basal body temperature to avoid pregnancy. If you see your temperature rising higher than usual or rising earlier than expected (whether or not you are feeling ill), you need to watch this unexpected temperature change carefully. If a fever is present, your temperature should be taken with a fever thermometer once in the morning and once in the evening until the fever is no longer present. A fever thermometer should be used since it measures the body temperature up to 108°F. The basal body temperature only goes up to 100°F. You will not be able to know how high your fever actually is if you use your basal body thermometer. It could also break if it is used to try to measure unusually high temperatures.

The unusually high temperature should be recorded on the fertility awareness chart in a special way each day it is present. If the temperature is higher than the temperatures printed on the chart (the chart goes up to 99°F), a line should be drawn from the last normal basal body temperature to the very top of the chart. Each day the temperature remains off the chart, it should be recorded in the "Notes" column. When you begin to recover from the illness, the basal body temperature will return to a normal level. You should then resume taking your temperature with the basal body thermometer and record it as usual.

When you have an illness that causes a fever, one of three situations may occur during the menstrual cycle:

1. Ovulation will occur as usual and the menstrual cycle will be its usual length.

2. Ovulation will occur later than usual and the menstrual cycle will be longer than its usual length.

3. Ovulation will not occur and bleeding may or may not be experienced. Even if this bleeding takes place around the time you would expect to see menstrual bleeding, do not consider this a true menstrual period.

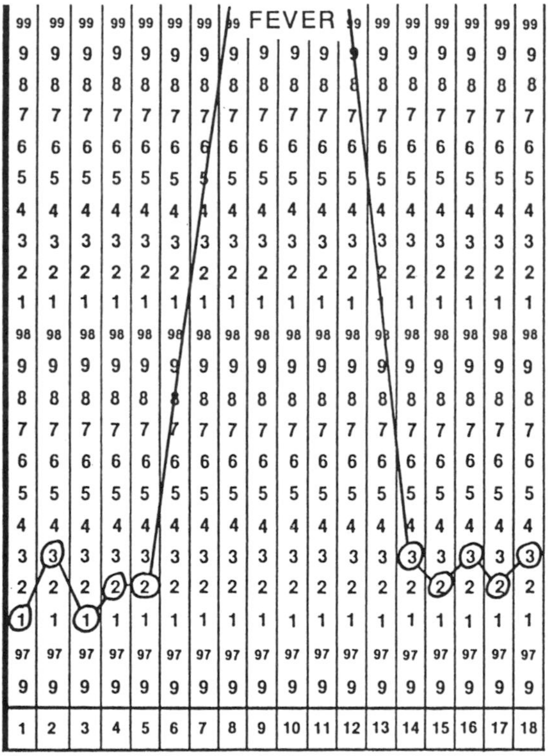

Figure 38 Charting a fever

In Figure 38, Sue began observing and recording her basal body temperature from the first day of her menstrual cycle. From cycle day 6 through cycle day 13 she experienced a fever above 99.1°F. She noted the presence of a fever on her chart. When the fever subsided, she resumed observing and recording her basal body temperature.

OVULATION ON TIME

When the high temperature from illness occurs during the time of ovulation, a thermal shift cannot be seen. However, you will know if you ovulate because, once the fever is gone, the temperature will drop back down to the high temperatures you normally experience after ovulation.

Observe your mucus during the fever. If the Peak Day Rule can be applied, you can follow this rule to determine when the infertile phase has begun. However, if you are not confident using this rule alone, you should wait until the Thermal Shift Rule can also be applied to be sure ovulation has taken place and the infertile phase after ovulation has begun.

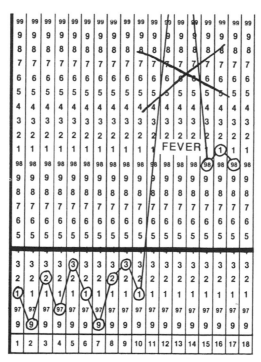

Figure 39 Fever during time of ovulation

In Figure 39, Alice experienced a fever from cycle day 11 through cycle day 15. Once the fever subsided, her basal body temperature was at the normal level experienced after ovulation. This indicated that ovulation had taken place at some point during the fever. To determine the infertile phase, she drew a coverline above the first ten normal low temperatures recorded before the fever.

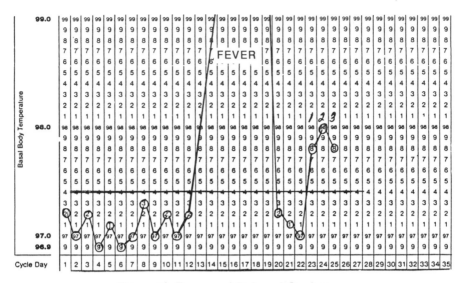

Figure 40 Fever and Delayed Ovulation

In Figure 40, Elisa usually has menstrual cycles ranging from 28–32 days. During a cycle when she was ill, she experienced ovulation later than was usual for her. This was seen by the fact that when her fever subsided on cycle day 20, her basal body temperature was still low. On cycle day 23 her temperature shifted and she was then able to apply the Thermal Shift Rule to determine her infertile phase.

LATE OVULATION

Ovulation may be delayed during an illness. A delayed ovulation is one that happens later than usual during the menstrual cycle. With a delayed ovulation the thermal shift may not be seen until a few days to a week later than usual. If ovulation did not occur during the fever, once it subsides the temperatures will return to the normal low level experienced before ovulation. In this situation, the woman should continue to take her BBT until the Thermal Shift Rule can be applied.

NO OVULATION

No ovulation is called *anovulation*. You may not ovulate at all during the time of illness.

Basal body temperature patterns during the anovulatory cycle

When ovulation does not occur, you will continue to experience a low temperature pattern. This low pattern is just like the one you normally see before ovulation. The thermal shift does not occur. In other words, since ovulation has not taken place, you are unable to apply the Thermal Shift Rule. However, you will be able to use your mucus observations, with special rules discussed later in this chapter, to avoid pregnancy.

Cervical mucus patterns during the anovulatory cycle

When ovulation does not occur, there is no one special pattern of mucus.

— You may produce mucus that remains sticky, pasty, and crumbly throughout the entire time you do not ovulate.

— You may not produce any mucus and remain dry at the outside of your vaginal area.

— You may experience wet mucus and a wet feeling at the outside of your vaginal area. The mucus may be of the creamy, wet type or may even feel somewhat slippery and stretchy. However, the mucus will not become the very wet, stretchy, and slippery type that occurs with ovulation.

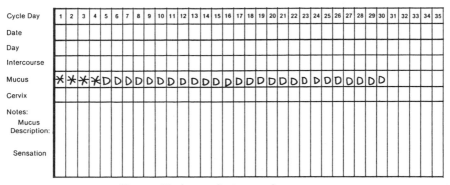

Figure 41 Anovulation and no mucus

In Figure 41, Jeanine had the flu one cycle, causing a time of anovulation. During the entire time she did not ovulate, mucus was not produced and a continuous dry vaginal sensation was present.

— You may experience a combination of these changes. For example, you may have dry days and sticky, pasty, and crumbly mucus days during the entire time you do not ovulate. Or you may experience sticky, pasty, and crumbly mucus days, totally dry days, and wet days during the entire time you do not ovulate.

Cervical Changes During the Anovulatory Cycle

— You may experience a low, firm, and closed cervix while you are not ovulating.

— You may experience a slightly raised, slightly soft, and slightly open cervix while you are not ovulating.

— You may even experience a combination of both, low to slightly high, firm to slightly soft, and closed to slightly open.

If you do not ovulate, you may or may not bleed, or spotting of blood may occur. If you do experience bleeding, it may be lighter or heavier than normal, and it may last shorter or longer than your usual menstrual bleeding. The important thing to remember is that *if bleeding of any type occurs during the times of anovulation, it is not menstrual bleeding. It could be a warning that ovulation is taking place or is going to take place. Therefore, any bleeding is treated as though it is mucus. It is a fertile time!*

We have given several possibilities for changes in fertility signs during the anovulatory cycle because a woman can experience a range of changes during times of anovulation.

Though this may be confusing for some women, when they observe their fertility signs carefully, they can provide themselves with an effective means of family planning.

Anovulation = No Ovulation = A Time of Temporary Infertility

SECONDARY SIGNS AND PREMENSTRUAL SIGNS

If you usually experience bodily changes which alert you to the approach of ovulation and your menstrual flow, they may be different or you may not experience them at all during the time that ovulation does not occur.

Temporary infertility means that fertility can return at any time. Since there isn't a way to predict when ovulation will return, the following special circumstances rules must be followed carefully when you question whether or not you are experiencing either delayed ovulation or anovulation. Since these rules will allow you to be on the lookout for signs of returning fertility, they will protect you against pregnancy.

Special Circumstances Rules

These rules are applied to the mucus observations when experiencing anovulation or delayed ovulation. *If properly followed, they can enable a woman to have intercourse safely while still being able to observe any mucus changes that could mean ovulation is approaching and therefore a return of fertility.*

> ### SPECIAL CIRCUMSTANCES RULE NUMBER 1
>
> ### Dry Day Rule: Intercourse can take place the night of a dry day

The **Dry Day Rule** states that intercourse may safely occur on the night of any dry day. A dry day means a day of no mucus and a dry vaginal sensation. The day after intercourse may be an

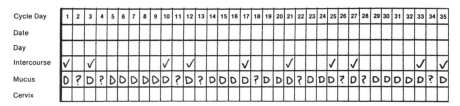

Figure 42 Use of the Dry Day Rule and Anovulation

In Figure 42, Diane has not ovulated for two months. Because she has experienced continuous dry days, she has used the Dry Day Rule whenever she has had intercourse. She had to abstain on the days after intercourse because she observed a vaginal discharge on these days (noted with a "?").

abstinence day if a vaginal discharge is observed. If semen is present in the vagina the day after intercourse, you will not know if mucus is present and if ovulation is going to take place. Intercourse can con tinue on the night of dry days throughout the time of anovulation.

SPECIAL CIRCUMSTANCES RULE NUMBER 2

Mucus Patch Rule: Abstinence from intercourse should be followed if one or more days of any type of mucus occurs after a dry day

and

If the mucus is pasty, sticky, or crumbly with a dry vaginal sensation, abstinence should be followed for two dry days after the mucus is no longer present

or

If the mucus is of a wet quality with a wet vaginal sensation, abstinence should be followed for 4 dry days after the mucus is no longer present

The **Mucus Patch Rule** states that if, following a dry day, you experience one day or more of any type of mucus and/or wet vaginal sensations, you must abstain from intercourse. The mucus or wet sensations could mean that ovulation is approaching.

If the mucus is sticky, pasty, and crumbly, and vaginal sensations are dry, you need to abstain during those days when the mucus is present and for 2 dry days after the mucus goes away. Then you can resume applying the Dry Day Rule.

If the mucus feels wet and vaginal sensations are wet, you need to abstain during those days when the mucus is present and for 4 dry days after the wet mucus goes away. Then you can resume applying the Dry Day Rule.

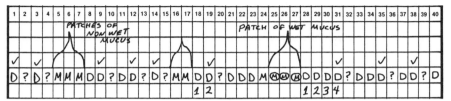

Figure 43 Use of the Dry Day Rule and Mucus Patch Rule
during Anovulation

In Figure 43, Morgan has been using the Dry Day Rule for the past 35 days. One day while checking for mucus, she notices the presence of sticky, pasty mucus. Since this could be a sign of approaching ovulation, she begins to abstain. She finds that she has 3 days of the sticky mucus and then returns to experiencing completely dry days. In this situation, Morgan abstains during the 3 days of mucus and for 2 dry days after the mucus ends. Because she did not ovulate, she resumes using the Dry Day Rule until mucus is again produced.

Morgan continues to use the Dry Day Rule on dry days and the Mucus Patch Rule during pasty, sticky mucus days. One day she notices a wet vaginal sensation and observes wet-feeling mucus. Since ovulation may be near, she abstains during the time when mucus is present. Once the mucus ends, she continues to abstain for 4 dry days instead of 2 dry days. This is because the mucus is wet and ovulation may have occurred. After applying the Mucus Patch Rule, she can resume using the Dry Day Rule during her completely dry days.

TO REVIEW

- Intercourse can occur the night of dry days.

- Abstinence should be followed during any days of mucus. If the mucus is crumbly, pasty, and sticky, abstinence continues until the evening of the second dry day after this mucus ends. If the mucus is wet, abstinence continues until the evening of the fourth dry day after the wet mucus ends.

THE BASIC INFERTILE PATTERNS OF CERVICAL MUCUS

During the times when a woman is not ovulating she may experience what is called a basic infertile pattern of cervical mucus. This means that instead of experiencing mostly dry days, *she experi-*

ences the same type of cervical mucus every day. Usually this non-changing mucus is the pasty, sticky mucus that doesn't feel wet. Another non-changing pattern is a slightly wet, creamy type of mucus. The non-changing, non-wet mucus days are treated as though they were dry days. In other words, because you experience continuous non-changing, non-wet mucus days instead of dry days, you can have intercourse every other non-changing mucus day. However, if you experience any change in the basic infertile pattern (a change in the mucus), you need to abstain because you may be approaching ovulation. To prevent pregnancy in this situation, the **Mucus Patch Rule** should be used. The Mucus Patch Rule for the basic infertile mucus pattern states that *abstinence should begin as soon as there is any change in the quality of the basic infertile mucus and should continue throughout the changing mucus and for 4 days after it ends.* If it does not become the very wet, stretchy, slippery mucus of ovulation and/or the Thermal Shift Rule cannot be applied, then ovulation probably did not occur. In this situation, intercourse can be resumed after the mucus has returned to the basic infertile mucus pattern for 4 days in a row. Then the Dry Day Rule is used until another mucus patch is observed.

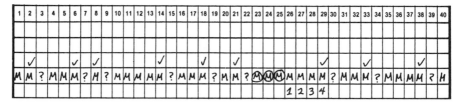

Figure 44 Use of the Dry Day Rule and Mucus Patch Rule with a
basic infertile mucus pattern

In Figure 44, Marlene has been experiencing anovulation for 3 months. During this time she has observed sticky, pasty, and non-wet mucus day after day, so she has been using the Dry Day Rule. One day she notices the mucus has changed. It now feels wet. This could be a sign of the approach of ovulation. Because of this she abstains during the days of the wet mucus. As soon as the mucus has returned to its basic infertile pattern of the non-wet, sticky, and pasty type for 4 days in a row, she can resume using the Dry Day Rule.

TO REVIEW

- Intercourse can occur the night of every other non-changing mucus day (Dry Day Rule)

- If the mucus changes, the Mucus Patch Rule is applied

- Once the Mucus Patch Rule has been applied, the Dry Day Rule can again be used

- Abstinence should be followed during any days of changing mucus

If any type of bleeding occurs during a time of anovulation, these days are treated as though they are wet mucus days. Bleeding can mean ovulation. However, bleeding makes it difficult to observe mucus accurately, therefore abstinence should be followed during any days of bleeding and for 4 days of the basic infertile pattern after the bleeding ends. If ovulation takes place during bleeding, you will see a thermal shift at this time.

CAUSES OF ANOVULATION

Although anovulation may last for a varied period of time, ovulation will usually return. When it does, you will observe the thermal shift and the very wet, slippery, stretchy mucus. The Thermal Shift Rule and Peak Day Rule can then be applied to determine the beginning of the infertile phase after ovulation.

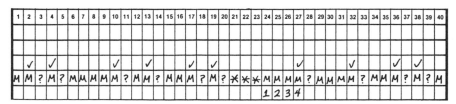

Figure 45 Anovulation, Mucus Patch and bleeding

In Figure 45, during the fourth month of anovulation, Marlene experiences bleeding. Since this could mean ovulation is occurring, she abstains during the bleeding. As soon as the mucus has returned to its basic infertile pattern for 4 days after the bleeding ends, she can resume using the Dry Day Rule.

Once ovulation returns, you can use the Menses and Dry Day Rules. Remember that the menstrual cycles may change after a period of anovulation. Therefore, it is important to observe six cycles before applying the Twenty-one Day Rule.

Anovulation has many causes. An illness with a fever is just one; some other causes include:

Illness

Some women's reproductive systems are greatly affected by any type of illness. Ovulation can stop because of an illness but will usually return once the illness is over.

Birth Control Pills

Birth control pills work to prevent pregnancy primarily by stopping ovulation. Once you stop taking them, ovulation may begin within 2–3 weeks or may not begin for a month or more. Even if ovulation begins right away and a thermal shift is observed, it may take a month or more for the mucus to return to a normal ovulatory mucus pattern. In other words, some women see a thermal shift, but the mucus does not seem to become the very wet, slippery, stretchy mucus. Because of this the Peak Day Rule cannot be applied. If this occurs, the Thermal Shift Rule can be used alone with a minimal possibility of pregnancy.

Change in Diet and/or Exercise Routine

When a woman changes her eating habits and/or exercise routine, she usually experiences a change in her body weight. Sometimes a 5–10-pound weight gain or loss can cause a change in the ovulatory pattern or can cause anovulation. A change in diet and/or exercise without a weight loss or gain can also have the same effect. Once the body becomes adjusted to this change in weight or change in exercise, ovulation usually returns.

Menopause

As a woman approaches her late 30s to her 40s, she will usually experience gradual changes in her menstrual cycle. She may not ovulate every month, or may ovulate every 2–3 months or even less frequently. After one full year of no menstrual bleeding, the possibility of ovulating is small. Once the full year has passed, a woman has reached the menopausal period of her life. Since a woman approaching menopause may ovulate infrequently, she should use the Dry Day and Mucus Patch Rules during the times of anovulation. When she does ovulate, she can apply the Thermal Shift and Peak Day Rules to determine the infertile phase after ovulation. A woman ovulating infrequently should not use the Twenty-one Day Rule. Therefore, the days of menstrual bleeding following ovulation would be considered fertile. Once the bleeding ends, she can resume the use of the Dry Day Rule and Mucus Patch Rule until she ovulates and the infertile phase after ovulation rules can be applied.

Emotional Stress

The way you feel emotionally can affect your body physically. Over the past few years the relationship of the mind and body has been studied to a great extent. It is well known that emotional stress can cause ulcers, backaches, and headaches. All of us experience stressful events in our lives: changing jobs, a death in the family, travel, family visits, and on and on. Any of these may cause you to not ovulate for a month or more.

Development of an Ovarian Cyst

Occasionally, the developing follicle may not continue to the point of ovulation. Instead it enlarges to form a cyst on the ovary, lasting about 2–6 weeks. Usually ovulation does not occur while the cyst is present. During this time irregular bleeding may be experienced or the menstrual period can be delayed a week or more.

Again, as with all other causes of delayed ovulation and anovulation, the Dry Day Rule and Mucus Patch Rule are used.

Breastfeeding

During breastfeeding, ovulation may occur irregularly or not at all. This usually depends upon the way you choose to breastfeed.

If you breastfeed throughout the day, each and every time the baby is hungry, or when the baby just desires the comfort of suckling at the mother's breast, there is a small chance of ovulation. This is because the pituitary gland, the small gland at the base of the brain, produces a hormone that stops ovulation. The amount of the hormone produced depends upon the number of times a day the baby is breastfed.

If you give the baby water, juice, or other types of nourishment, as well as allowing the baby to suck on a pacifier, you have a greater chance of ovulating. In this case it is important to always observe your fertility signs carefully. This is especially true when you stop feeding the baby at night or if anything else occurs which leads to the baby feeding at the breast less often.

The decision of how and why to breastfeed will depend upon many factors, including whether you are working or involved in other activities which prevent you from being with the baby throughout the day. Unfortunately, some women have been told that if they breastfeed once or twice a day, they will not ovulate and cannot become pregnant. This is not true. The return of ovulation is affected by the amount of suckling that occurs throughout the day. The less often the baby has an opportunity to suckle at the breast each day, the greater the chance of ovulation.

The return of ovulation, and therefore fertility, will vary from woman to woman. In general, the earliest return of ovulation for a woman who is totally breastfeeding is about 10 weeks after delivery. The *average* return of ovulation for a woman who is totally breastfeeding is about 14½ months after delivery. When bottle-feeding the baby, ovulation can begin within 2–4 weeks after delivery. The return of ovulation will depend partially upon when supplementary feeding is introduced, as well as when and how weaning of the baby begins. When fertility returns, the clear slippery mucus with a true, wet vaginal sensation, the shift in temperature, and a high, soft, and open cervix will be observed.

In general, a woman who is breastfeeding may experience one or more of these mucus patterns:

1. She may be completely dry, with no mucus during the entire time of total breastfeeding.

2. She may experience one or more days of crumbly, pasty, sticky mucus between dry days.

3. Occasionally a totally breastfeeding woman may also experience wet sensations and wet mucus, usually of the more creamy type. This type of mucus can be present between dry days or days of crumbly, pasty, sticky mucus.

4. After the weaning process begins, a woman is apt to notice an increase in the number of days when she experiences some type of mucus. As suckling is reduced, the body will increasingly try to ovulate until it succeeds. During this process the woman can experience a greater number of days of wet, somewhat slippery mucus.

5. Days of bleeding may even occur. Since mucus can be mixed in with the blood, *it is very important to treat the days of bleeding—even slight spotting—as fertile mucus days and to abstain from intercourse.*

The breastfeeding woman who is either not ovulating or ovulating occasionally needs to follow the Dry Day and Mucus Patch Rules. If you are interested in learning more about total breastfeeding and how to prolong anovulation, we suggest reading *Natural Breastfeeding and Childspacing* by Sheila Kippley. (See the Bibliography for this book and other books on breastfeeding.)

As with women experiencing anovulation for other reasons, observation of the cervix can prove helpful.

Some women who breastfeed and some women approaching menopause experience an extremely dry feeling in the vaginal canal. The loss of the usual moisture in these tissues is due to a lack of the estrogen that was usually present in large amounts with ovulatory cycles. If the vaginal tissues become dry, intercourse and urination can be uncomfortable or painful. A woman should talk with her doctor if this change in the vagina takes place.

Moist vaginal tissue helps cervical mucus travel down to the vaginal opening. Dry vaginal tissue does not aid the flow of mucus. A woman in this situation may find it helpful to use internal checking in combination with external checking. For example, the woman approaching menopause who experiences this type of premenopausal dryness may benefit from checking for mucus that may be present at the opening of the cervix. If the woman in this situation experiences a dry vaginal sensation and no mucus with external checking, yet with internal checking observes the presence of wet mucus, she should continue to check internally. Her dry vaginal tissue is slowing down the flow of wet mucus, therefore internal checking may be more effective for her.

How to Check for Mucus Internally:

1. Insert 2 fingers into the vagina until you feel the cervix

2. Place one finger on each side of the cervix

3. Gently press your fingers against the cervix

4. Move your fingers to the opening of the cervix to collect mucus

5. Remove your fingers and slowly stretch them apart

6. Observe the amount, color, and quality of the mucus

A word about basal body temperature for new mothers, women approaching menopause, and all other women experiencing anovulation: We realize that taking the basal body temperature every day may not be convenient. If the temperature cannot be taken every day, we strongly suggest taking it as soon as there is an appearance of wet mucus or a change in the basic infertile pattern. If the thermal shift occurs when there has been a mucus pattern that changes to ovulatory, wet, stretchy mucus, the Thermal Shift and Peak Day Rules can be applied to determine the beginning of the infertile phase after ovulation. However, until a woman has resumed ovulating for six cycles in a row, the Twenty-one Day Rule cannot be applied.

For example, Carmen has ovulated for the first time after one year of breastfeeding. She is now able to use the Thermal Shift and Peak Day Rules. Yet until her fertility signs give proof of ovulation for six cycles, she would consider herself fertile during any type of bleeding and would continue to use the Dry Day Rule and Mucus Patch Rule until the beginning of the infertile phase after ovulation.

You will be able to recognize anovulation and prevent pregnancy through careful observation of fertility signs. Missing periods for a few months in no way harms the body. However, if a woman has not experienced periods for more than 3 months for reasons other than total breastfeeding, we suggest that she discuss this situation with her doctor.

TO REVIEW

Basal Body Temperature

- A woman who ovulates will see her temperature shift from low to high

- A woman who does not ovulate will not see her temperature shift from low to high

Cervical Mucus

- A woman who ovulates will develop very wet, slippery, stretchy mucus as she approaches ovulation

- A woman who does not ovulate will not develop the true wet, stretchy mucus. She can experience a variety of mucus patterns from all dry days to a combination of wet-feeling mucus, pasty, sticky mucus, and dry days throughout the entire time she does not ovulate

Cervical Changes

- A woman who ovulates will experience a cervix that rises to a high position, becomes soft, and opens wide

- A woman who does not ovulate will experience a cervix that either remains low, firm, and closed or that rises slightly and becomes slightly soft and slightly open

Secondary Fertility Signs

- A woman who ovulates will notice one sign or more which shows she is ovulating

- A woman who is not ovulating will probably not experience her usual secondary fertility signs

Remember, if you have anovulatory cycles that continue beyond 3 months, it is important to discuss this with your physician. It is also helpful to take all of your fertility awareness charts to the physician as they can help him/her to better understand your particular situation.

OTHER SPECIAL CIRCUMSTANCES

After Childbirth

If you are not breastfeeding, you may begin ovulating within two weeks after the delivery. If you want to use your fertility signs to prevent pregnancy, you should begin observing your mucus and temperature as soon after the delivery as possible. It can be difficult for you to observe your fertility signs if you are a new mother, awakening at irregular times to take care of your new baby, etc. However, you should try to begin checking your mucus and cervix when the discharge from childbirth has stopped. This discharge is called **lochia**, and it can be very difficult, if not impossible, to check mucus with this discharge present. Usually, three weeks after delivery the lochia has stopped and observation of the mucus and cervix can begin. Also, by that time you should begin observing your temperature.

Vaginal Infection

Another common special circumstance is a vaginal infection. One of the symptoms of a vaginal infection is the presence of a discharge from the vagina that looks different from the normal vaginal and cervical secretions. The second symptom can be an odor in the vaginal area that is unlike the usual vaginal scent. A third symptom can be burning and/or itching in the vaginal area. If you experience one or more symptoms, it is important for you to be examined to identify the cause of the infection and receive proper treatment.

During the time of a vaginal infection you will have difficulty observing your mucus changes, particularly if you are using a medication in the form of a vaginal cream or suppository. However, you can still continue to take your basal body temperature. It is not advisable to check your cervix or have intercourse until the vaginal infection has cleared up. If the infection is healed by the time you have accurately applied the Thermal Shift Rule, you can safely resume intercourse.

Premenstrual Syndrome

Premenstrual Syndrome (PMS) is the name given to various troubling emotional and/or physical changes experienced by many women, lasting anywhere from 1–14 days, usually before menstruation begins. (Some women also seem to experience the changes only during menstruation and for a couple of days after menstruation ends.)

There are over 100 different signals known as premenstrual symptoms that let a woman know she is approaching the time of menstrual bleeding. The most common of these symptoms are nervous tension, mood swings, irritability, anxiety, headache, craving for sweets, increased appetite, heart pounding, fatigue, dizziness or fainting, depression, forgetfulness, crying, confusion, insomnia, weight gain, swelling of hands, feet and legs, breast tenderness, and abdominal bloating.

Research conducted about PMS has shown that this problem may be due to an imbalance in estrogen and progesterone. Some women with PMS have an abnormally high amount of estrogen combined with a normal or abnormally low amount of progesterone.

Regardless of the amounts of estrogen and progesterone a woman has, an imbalance in these hormones appears to affect the brain and other parts of the body. For example, some believe that the brain puts out abnormal amounts of special chemicals that affect the way a woman thinks and feels as well as contribute to the body's tendency to "hold water."

We could go on and discuss other research that has recently begun, research related to brain and body chemistry that might end up unraveling at least some of the causes of PMS. However, it is too early to draw any conclusions. Therefore, we are more concerned with the important question women are asking, "What can a woman do to help herself?" Another question to address is, "Does PMS affect the use of NFP and FAM?"

Does PMS Affect the Use of NFP and FAM?

Picture the woman who has applied the infertile phase rules to enable her to know when the egg is dead and gone. She resumes having intercourse or puts her method of birth control away, only to find that within a few days after ovulation she begins to experience breast tenderness, bloating, headaches, and fatigue? Does she now feel like having intercourse? Perhaps not! In other words, the woman following NFP or FAM who experiences PMS may have an infertile phase after ovulation partially or totally filled with physical and/or emotional changes that cause her to not want to engage in any kind of sexual activity. What then does the infertile phase after ovulation have to offer her if she is unable to use it?

In addition to how the woman feels, her fertility signs may show the results of PMS. We have observed slow rising temperature patterns, irregular mucus patterns, and temperatures which do not stay up for 12–16 days in some women with PMS. Whether the patterns of fertility signs are slightly or severely irregular due to PMS in every woman that has it is something no one knows. However, what *is* known is that a woman can help herself so that she can feel better, and if her fertility signs are affected, they will probably be easier to identify if her PMS is being treated successfully.

Treating PMS

It is quite common for some women to experience physical and emotional changes from caffeine, sugar, alcohol, and salt in their diets. Most women can begin to help themselves by following these nutritional guidelines:

— Limit eating refined sugar to 5 tablespoons a day (if you *have* to eat sugar)

— Limit alcohol to 1 oz. a day (if you *have* to drink an alcoholic beverage)

— Do not drink more than 1 cup of coffee or tea or an 8 oz. can of a soft drink with caffeine a day

— Limit tobacco use

— Limit intake of red meat to 3 oz. a day

— Rely more on fish, poultry, whole grains, and legumes as sources of protein and less on red meat and dairy products

— Eat leafy green vegetables and fresh fruit every day

— Use 2 tablespoons uncooked safflower oil on salads or vegetables every day

These guidelines for exercise and relaxation can also help:

— Take a 20-minute walk every day. Walking is a non-stress exercise that can build up strength, be relaxing, and get you out in the fresh air on a regular basis.

— If there is considerable stress in your life, deciding on a way to help decrease the stress can help. For example, talking with a counselor or therapist, meditating, listening to music, taking up a hobby, etc. A woman can benefit greatly from learning what helps her to relax and handle stressful situations better.

Many women also often benefit greatly from taking vitamins and minerals. Some research has shown that estrogen and progesterone may not be present in normal amounts because a woman's diet is lacking an adequate amount of all the B vitamins and magnesium.[4] Dr. Guy Abraham, a gynecologist and researcher of premenstrual problems for the past thirteen years, suggests following a well-balanced *total* vitamin and mineral program to help relieve premenstrual symptoms. Women with mild symptoms may need only one-half the amounts of the vitamins and minerals listed here. Women with moderate to severe symptoms would probably benefit by taking the full amounts.[5]

Vitamins	
Vitamin A	12,500 IU
Vitamin E (d-alpha tocopherol acid succ.)	100 IU
Vitamin D-3 (cholecalciferol)	100 IU
Folic Acid	200 mcg
Vitamin B-1 (thiamine mononitrate)	25 mg
Vitamin B-2 (riboflavin)	25 mg
Niacinamide	25 mg
Vitamin B-6	300 mg
Vitamin B-12	62.5 mcg
Biotin	62.5 mcg
Pantothenic acid	25 mg
Inositol	25 mg
Choline Bitartrate	312.5 mg
Para-amino benzoic acid	25 mg
Bioflavonoids	250 mg
Vitamin C (ascorbic acid)	1500 mg
Rutin	25 mg

IU—International Units   mcg—micrograms   mg—milligrams
All the vitamins except Vitamins A, E, and D-3 should be taken in sustained release form

Minerals	
Calcium	125 mg
Magnesium	250 mg
Iodine	75 mcg
Iron	15 mg
Copper	0.5 mg
Zinc	25 mg
Manganese	10 mg
Potassium	47.5 mg
Selenium	100 mcg
Chromium	100 mcg

All minerals should be taken in chelated form.
In addition, it is helpful to add digestive enzymes to aid the body in absorbing vitamins and minerals. These enzymes include:

Amylase Activity	15,000 USP units
Protease Activity	15,000 USP units
Lipase Activity	1,200 USP units
Betaine Acid HCL	100 mg

It is felt that the B-vitamins and all the other vitamins and minerals work together to help the liver break down estrogen and sugar. When these are broken down and used well by the body, the imbalance of various hormones may be reduced.

TIPS ON VITAMINS AND MINERALS

- Take them with a meal

- Take them every day

- Urine will probably be darker yellow in color and have a stronger than usual smell while you are taking them

- Intestinal gas can occur if a woman is not eating enough whole grains

- Vitamins and minerals work better if a woman is eating well, exercising regularly, and getting fresh air at least 20 minutes a day, four days a week

Progesterone therapy, as well as the use of various drugs, are other approaches to the treatment of PMS. Again, research is limited as to whether drugs and hormones really work for every woman with PMS. If a woman wishes to use progesterone or certain drugs, it is an extremely good idea to combine this drug therapy with a nutritional, exercise, and vitamin and mineral program. Remember to see the Bibliography for books that discuss PMS.

Some women have stated that when they have decreased the amount of mucus-producing foods (for example, dairy foods) in their diets, they have noticed a decrease in the amount of cervical mucus produced. Other women who have needed to take prescription antihistamines, drugs that dry up the secretions in the nasal passages, notice a drying up of their mucus.

You can become aware of the factors that might affect your own mucus pattern. If you change your diet or need to take certain drugs and see a change in your mucus pattern, with careful observation you will probably be able to utilize your mucus to avoid pregnancy. If you experience a substantial decrease in mucus or a constant dry feeling, yet you know you are ovulating by seeing a thermal shift, you may need to use internal checking. If you find yourself confused or concerned, talking with your doctor—as well as having a physical examination—will be helpful. It may also be valuable to seek advice from a fertility awareness instructor.

As you can see, just about every woman can observe her fertility signs as a means of pregnancy avoidance. If you experience a special circumstance, be on the lookout for signs of fertility and follow the rules carefully. Please remember that the language your body speaks is a clear, accurate language. The time and effort you spend will enable you to understand it. We hope you will be encouraged, for the language is worth the learning.

YOUR NOTES:

_____

_____

_____

_____

_____

_____

_____

_____

_____

Chapter 12

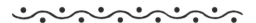

The Fertility Awareness Method

Some things catch on because they are fads; other ideas catch on because they are sound, valuable and workable.

The **Fertility Awareness Method** (FAM) is such a concept. Increasingly, couples are turning away from the Pill and the IUD, and using barrier and/or spermicidal methods. And some couples are turning away from barrier and/or spermicidal methods toward FAM. The reason for the change to FAM is both reasonable and simple.

It is reasonable because it is based on natural body awareness, and it is simple because the information you need to follow is always with you.

Couples who have been using barrier methods of birth control (condom, diaphragm, and cervical cap) and couples who have been using spermicides (jelly, creams, foam, and suppositories) *have an alternative, so they don't have to use these methods each time they have intercourse.* FAM is based on the same scientific principles as natural family planning, yet FAM is for those who do not wish to abstain from intercourse during the fertile days of the menstrual cycle. This means that only during fertile days is it necessary to use another method of birth control. Therefore, the number of days these methods are necessary can be greatly decreased.

Traditionally, men and women have learned that a contraceptive device must be used every time they have intercourse. This is not necessary, since the number of fertile days during each cycle averages from five to seven. A couple having intercourse during this time can use any of the methods mentioned above, and do not need to use any additional contraception during the infertile days. In other words, fertility awareness method offers choices and options in avoiding pregnancy. The options or variations you choose depend on the barrier and/or spermicidal method of birth control you wish to use and on the fertility signs you wish to observe.

The way in which FAM is used also depends upon how you feel about using the other methods of birth control. For example, Judy has been using the diaphragm for two years. Although she is basically satisfied with it, she and her partner have been talking about changing their method of birth control to one that does not interrupt their lovemaking. They feel that at times the diaphragm does not allow them the freedom they would like to have with intercourse. This couple decided to give FAM a chance, and Judy learned how to determine her fertile and infertile phases. Once she learned this, she and her partner no longer needed to use the diaphragm each time they had intercourse. Now that they need to use the diaphragm less often, they no longer feel the need to change their method of birth control.

How can you minimize the use of birth control methods after ovulation? We have already discussed the factors which can prevent you from accurately observing your cervical mucus. One of these factors is spermicidal preparations. These chemicals, when inserted into the vagina with or without the diaphragm, condom, or cervical cap, kill the sperm. They also cover up cervical mucus. Therefore, if you choose to use a spermicide, you will be unable to observe your mucus changes during the days when the spermicide is present in your vagina. However, the fertility sign which *can* be observed is your basal body temperature.

The basal body temperature can be used with or without cervical changes. Observation of the basal body temperature used with the application of the Thermal Shift Rule can provide you with a way to identify the infertile phase after ovulation. Once this phase begins, additional birth control is no longer necessary until the beginning of the next menstrual cycle.

For example, a woman can use contraceptive foam until she can apply the Thermal Shift Rule. Once the infertile phase begins,

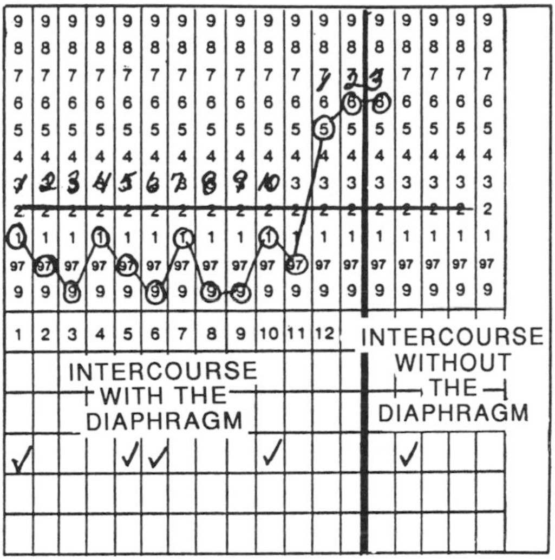

Figure 46 Diaphragm use and the Thermal Shift Rule

In Figure 46, Carmen did not want to use the Twenty-one Day Rule. Instead she used her diaphragm whenever she had intercourse until she determined she was no longer fertile. Because she was using the diaphragm, she chose to observe only her basal body temperature. By applying the Thermal Shift Rule she found that her postovulatory infertile phase began on the evening of cycle day 14. From that evening through the remainder of that menstrual cycle she could have intercourse safely without the need for her diaphragm.

---

she no longer needs to use the contraceptive foam for the remainder of that menstrual cycle. Knowing when the infertile phase after ovulation begins eliminates the need for birth control for about 10 days of the menstrual cycle.

Another example of how FAM can be applied is the use of the non-lubricated condom in combination with cervical mucus and basal body temperature observations. Because the condom prevents semen from entering the vagina, the cervical mucus is not affected. Use of the condom allows accurate observation of mucus changes and successful application of the Peak Day Rule. For instance, a couple may use the non-lubricated condom until the Thermal Shift and Peak Day Rules are applied to determine the beginning of the infertile phase after ovulation. Once this phase begins, the condom is not needed for the remainder of that menstrual cycle.

How can you minimize the use of birth control methods before ovulation? The Twenty-one Day Rule can be used just as it is in natural family planning to provide you with days for intercourse before ovulation that are very safe from pregnancy.

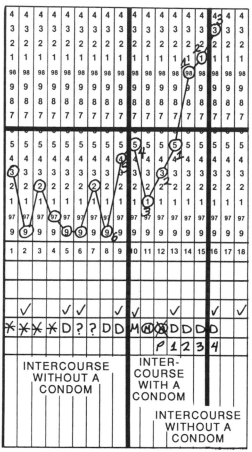

Figure 47 Condom use and the Twenty-one Day and Thermal Shift Rules

In Figure 47, Chris has a preovulatory infertile phase of 9 days. During that time she and Nick had intercourse without using a method of contraception. Since they wished to have intercourse after the start of the fertile phase on day 10, they used a non-lubricated condom. Use of the condom enabled them to observe the cervical mucus changes. They continued to use a condom until they could apply the Peak Day and Thermal Shift Rules. Once the infertile phase began on the evening of cycle day 16, they continued having intercourse, but without the need for a condom the remainder of that menstrual cycle.

Here are some typical cases:

If your last six menstrual cycles were 30, 31, 30, 29, 30, and 29 days long, by subtracting 21 from the shortest of the six cycles you have an infertile phase before ovulation of 8 days (29-21=8). The first 8 days of your menstrual cycle can be used to have intercourse without another method of birth control. When the fertile phase begins, and if you choose to have intercourse, you can utilize another method of birth control until you can successfully apply the Thermal Shift Rule (and if possible apply the Peak Day Rule). Once the infertile phase after ovulation begins, you no longer need to use your other method of birth control for the remainder of the menstrual cycle.

To reduce the pregnancy rate during the infertile phase before ovulation and the fertile phase, the Menses Rule and the Dry Day Rule can be used, as explained in Chapter 10. The Dry Day Rule can only be applied if you are able to check for the presence or absence of mucus. The non-lubricated condom is the only method that enables you to watch for the presence of early warning mucus, which could indicate an early ovulation.

As you can see, there are a variety of ways in which fertility signs, rules, and other methods of birth control can be combined to avoid pregnancy.

Contraceptive methods can be used during the fertile phase only, or during the infertile phase before ovulation and the fertile phase. It all depends on how great the desire is to avoid pregnancy and to decrease the use of another method of birth control.

As discussed in Chapter 2, it is generally believed that the pregnancy rates with FAM should not be any higher than the rates are when using the barrier and/or spermicidal methods alone, providing the rules are followed carefully.

Your willingness to observe your fertility signs and use the birth control methods conscientiously are the key to FAM. Because intercourse is taking place during the fertile phase—the phase with the highest risk of pregnancy—the careful and consistent use of the methods is of utmost importance if pregnancy is to be avoided.

Chapter 13

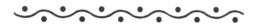

The Advantages and Disadvantages Of Natural Family Planning and Fertility Awareness Methods

The majority of this book has been about facts. Facts about the reproductive organs, the menstrual cycle, and fertility signs and rules. We hope what you have learned has been valuable for you and that you will be able to use all of these facts in many rewarding ways.

Knowing these facts can help you discover how you *feel* about yourself, your sexuality, and pregnancy. This is what this chapter is about: feelings ... feelings about fertility and sexuality, and what these feelings mean to you. This is of great importance, because your feelings will determine what the possible advantages and disadvantages of natural family planning will be for you.

SHOULD YOU USE NATURAL FAMILY PLANNING?

A conscious decision to use NFP, or any method of family planning for that matter, is one that only you can make. Taking time to personally examine the advantages and disadvantages of NFP will help you to answer the very important question of whether or not you should use it as your method of family planning.

Advantages ...

- NFP is not physically harmful.

- It promotes an understanding of the fertility cycle.

- It can be used by the woman who has truly irregular menstrual cycles, is breastfeeding, or is premenopausal.

- It is as effective in preventing pregnancy, if used properly, as most other birth control methods.

- It requires the man's cooperation and mutual sharing of responsibility for fertility control. NFP can promote a greater understanding of one another's sexual and emotional needs, and it can enhance a couple's love and respect for each other.

- In addition, it is an inexpensive means of family planning.

Disadvantages . . .

- NFP initially requires more time to learn and use than other family planning methods.

- It requires the cooperation of the man.

- It may require a change in sexual lifestyle, since abstinence during the fertile days is necessary.

- Because it requires more cooperation from the man, NFP is not used properly as often as the Pill and the IUD. Therefore, in actual use it is not as effective as the Pill and the IUD.

What may be experienced as an advantage for some may be a disadvantage for others. For example, if the man finds it difficult to abstain during the fertile days and is not supportive of fertility sign observation and charting, then the relationship may be disrupted. Or if the man wants to use NFP and the woman finds it difficult to abstain during the fertile days, likewise the relationship may be disrupted. However, when there is mutual commitment to abstinence, the relationship is often enhanced.

If you are considering NFP as a method of avoiding pregnancy, an important question to ask yourself is: Can I reach a mutual agreement with my partner to abstain from intercourse periodically and feel good about this way of avoiding pregnancy?

For some, this may be a difficult question. It can be helpful, when trying, to consider if in your relationship you are able to talk together openly and honestly about how to avoid pregnancy.

If your relationship is one in which effective and satisfying communication about sexuality and fertility control cannot occur, it does not mean it will always be that way. In a relationship a man and woman learn, grow, and change. And fortunately, there are ways to help the growing process so people can experience and enjoy the kinds of relationships they want.

With so many social changes taking place so rapidly in our society, there is a great opportunity for women and men to learn about themselves and their sexuality. This new awareness can enable them to make more responsible decisions than ever before.

WHAT DOES SEXUALITY MEAN?

For some, sexuality only means intercourse—an activity for the main purpose of babymaking. For others, it means a variety of ways of physical pleasuring. And for others, it has a different meaning, including more than sexual activity. This broader definition includes all of the physical and emotional aspects of being a man or a woman—the way a person walks, talks, dresses, makes love, the household duties a person chooses to do, as well as the type of job someone has.

Keeping this broader definition in mind, let's take a look at how we learn about sexuality. Learning about sexuality begins at birth and continues throughout our lifetime. This learning is influenced by everything and everyone around us. Unfortunately, much of the learning involves information that is usually incorrect or incomplete, and it often gives us messages that our genitals are "dirty" and that sex is something to be hidden. As children we tried to learn what sex was all about. Often this learning was done in "secret," behind the garage, in the attic, or in the basement. Then, as puberty approached, our bodies began to change. These changes, such as menstruation, breast development, sexual feelings, wet dreams, pubic hair, and acne, often created uncomfortable and frightening feelings.

Somehow, as if by magic, in adolescence we were expected to have healthy, mature attitudes about our bodies, our sexuality, and ourselves. Finally, as adults we are expected to be knowledgeable, sensitive, and comfortable about our sexuality, and to take responsibility for our sexuality and fertility. This is not easy when so many of us received a great deal of misinformation and many negative messages about our sexuality.

Misinformation and negative messages are major reasons why people either do not use birth control, or use it improperly. For example, a woman and man who are uncomfortable about their own sexuality often do not take responsibility for avoiding pregnancy, even though they are having intercourse. When an accidental pregnancy occurs, many women say, "I didn't know it (intercourse) was going to happen" or "I didn't think I could get pregnant." The man often says, "It was her fault. She should have done something to prevent the pregnancy."

Misinformation and negative messages not only contribute to unplanned pregnancies, they can also lead to sexual concerns and difficulties. These concerns include many types of dissatisfaction during lovemaking, from the woman who wants an orgasm but doesn't achieve one, to the man who is unable to have or keep an erection.

Other common reasons for sexual dissatisfaction are disagreements about the times to make love, how long it should last, and the type of sexual activity that occurs. For example, a woman may prefer sex in the morning, while her partner may prefer sex in the evening.

It is estimated that 9 out of 10 couples experience dissatisfaction at some time during their relationship because of a lack of accurate information about sex and the failure of the woman and man to communicate sexual feelings.

When uncertain of the facts about sex, people are often afraid to discuss it. Asking questions about sex and talking with a partner, doctor, friend, or counselor can be difficult. A person may fear sounding foolish or abnormal in some way. To some, talking with a partner means acknowledging unhappiness with their lovemaking. Because of this, a person may be afraid that his or her partner will feel hurt or become angry.

What we are saying is that there are very real reasons why people aren't open with their feelings. But this doesn't mean they shouldn't try. Once women and men begin to talk about their feelings, they are often amazed to find that their partners have many of the same questions and fears. By sharing these thoughts they become closer, which helps to enhance not only their sexual lives but other aspects of their relationship as well.

Many couples have also found that by talking, planning, and agreeing on how they want their sexual life to be, they set aside time for giving each other attention and pleasure.

DO YOU WANT A PREGNANCY?

This is one of the major questions related to fertility and sexuality that doesn't get asked or decided on as frequently as it should be. The answer to this question is determined by many factors, since people decide to have children for different reasons.

There are many reasons why people want children. Some of the reasons can be disruptive to the relationship, while others lead to the development of a loving and happy family.

— "To share our love with another human being"

— "We have so much to give"

— "A woman isn't a woman until she has a child"

— "A man isn't a man until he has a child"

— "To have someone to love"

— "To carry on the family name"

— "To give parents grandchildren"

— "It's normal and expected"

Some men and woman see a child as a solution to a problem in their lives.

— "Having a baby will keep us together"

— "Having a baby will keep my wife in her place"

— "Having a baby will make my husband happy, even if I don't want a child right now"

— "Nothing seems to help these lonely feelings I have"

— "I'm nothing unless I am a mother/father"

Having a child can be one of the most wonderful and gratifying experiences in life. Yet, the decision to have a child should not be taken lightly. It requires a great deal of thought, for it is about whether or not a couple have reached a time in their lives when they can care for and love each other, as well another human being.

Just as there are many reasons why people choose to have a child, there are also many reasons why couples choose to avoid having a child, at least for a period of time.

— "I can't provide for another person at this time in my life"

— "I feel emotionally fulfilled with the child/children I have"

— "Having a child right now would take time away from developing our relationship"

The decision to avoid a pregnancy or to become pregnant may be difficult to make. Yet, it must be made consciously if any method of birth control is to be used effectively.

When a couple have not firmly decided upon a birth control method, there are certain situations in which unplanned pregnancies frequently occur. These include a holiday, vacation, a romantic evening, and an occasion where drugs or alcohol are used. When people are relaxed and not feeling the stress in their lives, life's responsibilities and demands do not seem as great, and the desire for sexual pleasure can be increased. In these situations women often become pregnant, since at that time having a baby seems like the right thing to do. Unfortunately, after the vacation is over or the effects of the alcohol have worn off, the stresses of real life return, and the pregnancy is often viewed as a tragedy.

Not only do unplanned pregnancies occur frequently during these situations, they often result when a woman or man is experiencing major life changes. Such changes include a separation from a marriage or relationship, graduation from high school or college, dissatisfaction with a job or career, feelings of loneliness, or other times of unhappiness. Men and women have been known to think that having a child will be the answer to these problems.

We've discussed above some of the facts about sexuality, reasons people have for avoiding and achieving pregnancy, as well as many of the situations in life which commonly lead to pregnancy.

We feel (and perhaps you will agree) that fertility and sexuality play a major role in determining who we are and what we do. And as with all good things, sometimes there are problems. The reassuring point is that working out the problems can be a rewarding and positive experience.

HOW DOES NATURAL FAMILY PLANNING FIT INTO ALL OF THIS?

Many couples who make the choice to abstain from intercourse during the fertile days say that sharing in this method has been an enriching experience for their relationship. Many women not involved in a sexual relationship with one particular person find that using fertility signs to avoid pregnancy gives them a sense of control over their reproduction. They also find that when their partner learns more about how they avoid pregnancy, he is often fascinated by it, desires to learn more, and is supportive of the method.

By discussing their feelings, some men and women find that abstinence from intercourse—and even all sexual activity—during their fertile time works perfectly for them. Others discover that they chose to enjoy their partners sexually in ways other than intercourse.

Expressing sexuality without having intercourse brings other issues to mind about the use of NFP. Abstinence, in its true definition, means to not have intercourse. For some it also means to not experience other forms of sexual pleasuring, such as oral sex and other forms of sensual touching. For others it means that fertile days can be sexually enjoyable times without experiencing intercourse. It becomes a time for touching, massaging, caressing and enjoying any type of physical contact that a man and woman feel comfortable with. Others who find sexual contact—without intercourse—during fertile times difficult, frustrating, or against their beliefs, find that they are able to share love, affection, and enjoyable times without sexual activity.

In fact, it is sad to say—but great to know—that couples often experience a rebirth in their relationship when they can't have intercourse whenever they desire to. By "sad to say" we mean that it is not unusual for a couple to fall into a routine in which they forget to compliment each other, do things for one another and, in general, enjoy each other without sex. Women and men have commented that becoming aware of fertility and sharing the responsibility of birth control in their sexual relationship has given them a new view of their relationship and their reasons for being together—a new awakening, so to speak. For many, this new and greater understanding has enhanced their love for each other.

THE ADVANTAGES OF FERTILITY AWARENESS METHOD

The use of FAM involves all that we have discussed above, plus a bit more. Many couples feel that abstinence seems "unnatural" to them and isn't compatible with their lives. Others feel that if a fertile time coincides with a vacation, holiday, birthday, or just a day when the woman or man feels sexual, they want to be able to have intercourse, yet not want a pregnancy to result. Many are comfortable with the use of the diaphragm, condom, or spermicide and also feel that they benefit from not feeling "tied down" to these methods each time they have intercourse. FAM offers a choice for them.

A FEW LAST WORDS . . .

We hope that you have enjoyed *The Fertility Awareness Handbook* and through it have learned exciting, interesting, and helpful information. After reading about fertility, some people find that they wish to have the information reinforced for them or the opportunity to share particular questions and concerns with someone knowledgeable about the information. If you find this is true for you, there are various ways to locate such a person. One way is through a fertility awareness class. Though there may not be such classes in all areas of the country, by contacting a church group, your state department of public health, or a family planning or local planned parenthood organization, you can learn what in-structors and/or physicians are available to help you.

It is impossible in one short book about fertility awareness to provide all of the available information about sexuality, communi-cation, and relationships. However, we wanted to give you some "food for thought" and encouragement so that, if you haven't already, you will begin to do what is important for you—to feel that you are in control of your reproductive and sexual lives in ways that are best for you. We hope you will gain this control. We are discovering more and more that, regardless of age, type of rela-tionship, or how men and women choose to use fertility awareness information, it has enabled them to learn about themselves and each other.

Through this learning process couples are sharing feelings and mutual responsibility for enjoying their sexuality. They have learned to feel comfortable about the role fertility plays in their lives. We hope you will, too.

Sample NFP Contracts

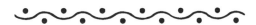

The thought of a birth control contract may sound cold and impersonal or perhaps even strange to you. Or it may be an exciting concept.

We've chosen to include it because some women and men have found that it helps them to talk with one another in order to make decisions concerning their sexual lives and feelings about pregnancy and birth control.

The nice part of the contract is that it is negotiable. This means that at any time the couple can change it! Let's say one of the partners in a relationship is feeling as though she/he wants to have a child, when six months ago that person felt quite the opposite. The contract can be "pulled out" and discussed, and perhaps changed. So a contract can be a helpful way to regularly assess one's personal needs.

Here are examples of two such contracts for use in natural family planning. If they don't quite suit your needs, feel free to adapt them or to write one of your own.

SAMPLE CONTRACT FOR THE WOMAN

I understand that if this method is to work, I must use it carefully and correctly.

Because I know that there are many reasons for taking chances and allowing pregnancy to happen, I will always explore, try to understand and, if I choose, communicate my feelings about what a pregnancy means to me.

I understand that to avoid a pregnancy means:

— No genital to genital contact (the penis cannot touch the vagina), and

— No intercourse during the fertile time.

Because I respect myself and am aware of my responsibility to myself, I agree to abide by this contract.

Should problems arise with the use of the method, or should I change my mind about avoiding pregnancy, I will decide how to best meet my needs and change the contract accordingly.

by: _____   _____

     Signature   Date

SAMPLE CONTRACT FOR THE COUPLE

We understand that if this method is to work, we must use it carefully and correctly.

Because we know that there are many reasons for taking chances and allowing a pregnancy to happen, we will always explore, try to understand, and communicate our feelings about what a pregnancy means to us.

We understand that to avoid a pregnancy means:

— No genital to genital contact (the penis cannot touch the vagina), and
— No intercourse during the fertile time.

Should problems arise with the use of the method, or should one of us change his/her mind about avoiding pregnancy, we will discuss this with each other and mutually agree upon how the contract should be changed.

by: _____   _____

     Signature   Date

by: _____   _____

     Signature   Date

Notes

1. Arthur Allbutt, *Wife's Handbook* (4th ed.; London: Forder, 1887)

2. Carl Gottfried Hartman, *Science and the Safe Period; a Compendium of Human Reproduction* (Baltimore: Williams and Wilkins, 1962).

3. Ibid.

4. Guy Abraham, M.D., "Premenstrual Tension," *Current Problems in Obstetrics and Gynecology III* August, 1980.

5. Ibid.

Bibliography
and List of References

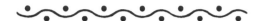

Since it is impossible for most people to "keep track" of the many new books related to fertility and sexuality being published today—much less read them all—we've listed a few that we thought might be of interest to you.

Abbot, Franklin. *Men and Intimacy.* Freedom, CA: The Crossing Press, 1990.

Abraham, Guy E., M.D. *Pre-Menstrual Blues.* Opitmox, P.O. Box 7000-280, Palos Verdes Peninsula, CA 90274, 1981.

Ammer, Christine. *The New A-to-Z of Women's Health: A Concise Encyclopedia.* Alameda, CA: Hunter House, 1991.

Barbach, Lonnie Garfield. *For Yourself.* New Jersey: Signet Books, 1976.

Blandau, R. and K. Moghissi. *The Biology of the Cervix.* Chicago: University of Chicago Press, 1973.

Bartzen, Peter, M.D. "Effectiveness of the Temperature Rhythm System of Contraception," *Fertility and Sterility.* Birmingham: American Fertility Association, 1967.

Berkeley Holistic Health Center. *The Holistic Health Handbook.* Berkeley: And/Or Press, 1978.

Billings, E.L. "Symptoms and Hormonal Changes Accompanying Ovulation," *The Lancet.* London: Little Brown and Co., February, 1972.

Billings, Evelyn, M.D. *The Billings Method.* New York: Ballantine, 1983.

Bing, Elizabeth. *Having a Baby Over 30.* New York: Bantam Books, 1978.

Borg, Susan and Judith Lasker. *When Pregnancy Fails.* New York: Beacon Press, 1981.

Boston Women's Health Book Collective. *The New Our Bodies, Ourselves.* New York: Simon and Schuster, 1984.

Boston Women's Health Book Collective. *Ourselves and Our Children.* New York: Random House, 1978.

Chopra, Deepak, M.D. *Quantum Feelings.* New York: Bantam Books, 1989.

Dalton, Katharina, M.D. *Once a Month: The Original Premenstrual Syndrome Handbook.* Fourth Edition. Claremont, CA: Hunter House, 1990.

DeVangelis, Barbara. *How to Make Love All the Time.* New York: Dell Publishers, 1988.

Hartman, Carl Gottfried. *Science and the Safe Period; a Compendium of Human Reproduction.* Baltimore: Williams and Wilkins, 1962.

Huggins, Kathleen. *The Nursing Mother's Companion.* Boston: Harvard Common Press, 1986.

Iffy, L., M.D. "Risks of Rhythm Method of Birth Control," *The Journal of Reproductive Medicine.* Chicago: Journal of Reproductive Medicine, September, 1970.

Kass-Annese, Barbara. *Say Goodbye to PMS.* New York: Warner Books, 1984.

Keefe, Edward F., M.D. "Self-Observation of the Cervix to Distinguish Days of Possible Fertility," *Bulletin of the Sloane Hospital for Women.* New York, 1962.

Kippley, J. *The Art of Natural Family Planning.* Cincinnati: Couple to Couple League, 1975.

Luker, K. *Taking Chances: Abortion and the Decision Not to Contracept.* Berkeley: University of California Press, 1975.

Madaras, Lynda et al., M.D. *Womancare: A Gynecological Guide to Your Body.* New York: Avon, 1981.

Marshall, John. "Cervical Mucus and Basal Body Temperature Method of Regulating Births—Field Trial," *The Lancet.* London: Little, Brown and Co., August 7, 1976.

Mayle, Peter. *What's Happening to Me?* Secaucus, NJ: Lyle Stuart, 1989.

——. *Where Did I Come From?* Secaucus, NJ: Lyle Stuart, 1990.

Menning, Barbara Eck. *Infertility, A Guide for the Childless Couple.* New York: Prentice Hall, 1988.

Ojeda, Linda. *Menopause Without Medicine.* Second Edition. Alameda, CA: Hunter House, 1992.

Raab, Diana. *Getting Pregnant and Staying Pregnant: Overcoming Infertility and Managing Your High Risk Pregnancy.* Alameda, CA: Hunter House, 1991.

Ratcliff, J.D. *Your Body and How It Works.* [n.p.]: Reader's Digest Press, Delacorte Press, 1975.

Ryder, Norman B. "Contraceptive Failure in the United States," *Family Planning Perspectives,* 5:133–142, 1973.

Segal, Jeanne, M.D. *Feeling Great: Enhancing Your Health and Well-Being.* Santa Cruz, CA: Unity Press, 1981.

Shivanandan, Mary. *Challenge to Love.* Bethesda, MD: KM Associates, 1988.

Trien, Susan Slamholtz. *Change of Life.* New York: Ballantine, 1986.

Vollman, R.F. *The Menstrual Cycle. Major Problems in Obstetrics and Gynecology.* v. 7 Philadelphia: Saunders, 1977.

Wade, Maclyn E., and others. "Use-Effectiveness of Two Methods of Natural Family Planning: An Interim Report," *American Journal of Obstetrics and Gynecology.* Boston: Boston, Massachusetts Medical Society, 1979.

Whelan, Elizabeth, ScD. *Boy or Girl?* New York: Pocket Books, 1978.

Index